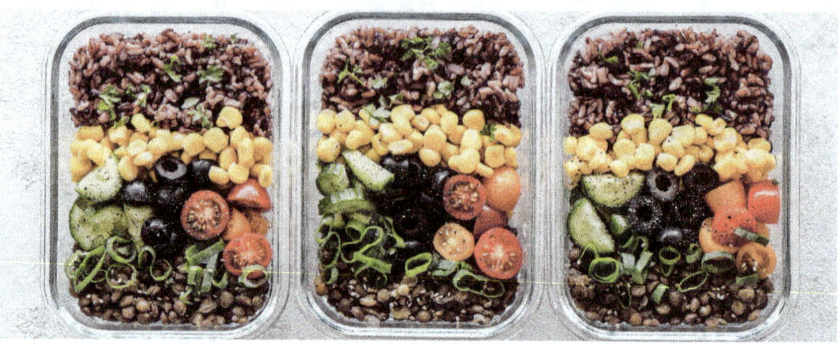

Introduction

Meal prep for nurses is a practical and efficient approach to maintaining a balanced diet amidst the demanding and often unpredictable schedules of the healthcare profession. With long shifts and little time for breaks, nurses can benefit significantly from planning and preparing their meals in advance. This not only ensures they have nutritious options readily available but also helps to reduce stress and save time during busy workdays. By incorporating meal prep into their routine, nurses can fuel their bodies properly, support their energy levels, and ultimately enhance their overall well-being while providing the best care to their patients.

Contents

01 The Nurse's Guide to Meal Prep Madness

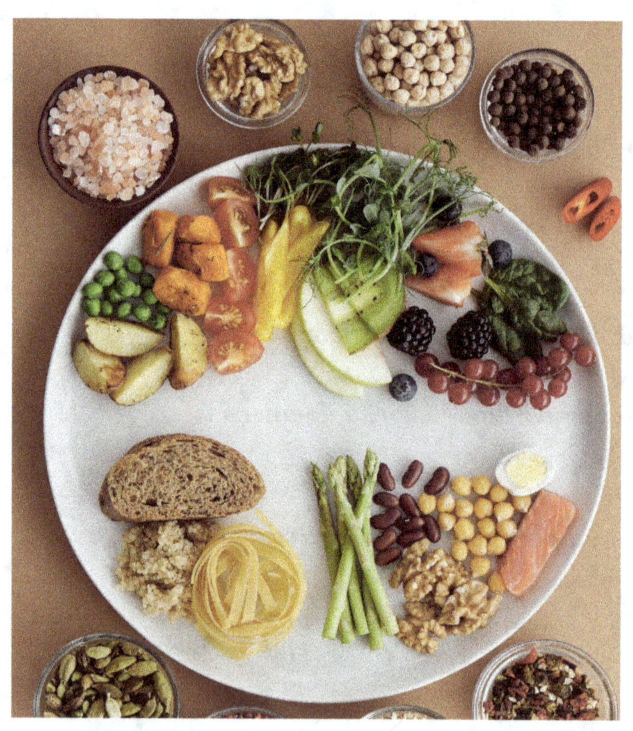

Why Meal Prep? Because Caffeine Can't Do It All!

Let's face it, caffeine is like that friend who promises to help you move but never actually lifts a finger when the time comes. You might think that a strong cup of coffee is all you need to power through those long shifts and chaotic days filled with demands, but let's be real - relying solely on caffeine is like trying to run a marathon in flip-flops. Sure, you might make it to the finish line eventually, but you'll be limping and struggling the entire way. Meal prep is your secret weapon in this scenario, ensuring you're not just barely surviving on liquid motivation but truly thriving on real nourishment that fuels your body and mind. By planning and preparing your meals in advance, you can set yourself up for success, making it easier to tackle whatever challenges come your way.

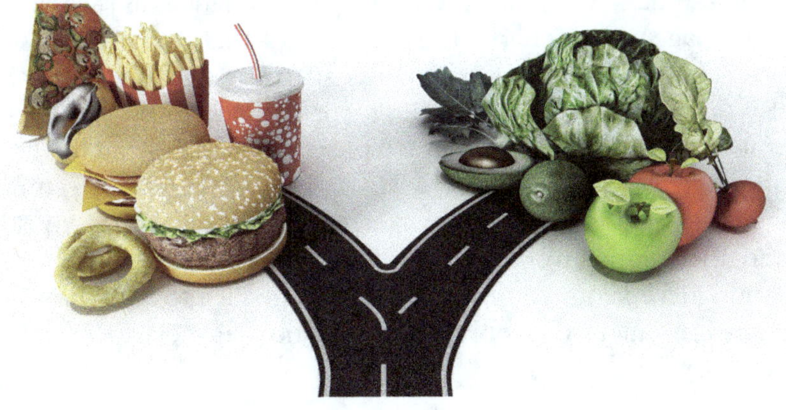

Picture this: you're halfway through a grueling 12-hour shift, your stomach growls louder than your patient's monitor, echoing through the sterile halls, and you suddenly realize that the only thing standing between you and a bag of stale chips is a lukewarm cup of coffee that barely touches the spot. Not exactly the kind of fuel you need when you're fighting the clock to save lives and keep your patients stable. By taking the time to plan ahead and prep your meals in advance, you can effectively avoid those desperate snack attacks that inevitably lead to regret (and a potential sugar crash at the most critical moment). Meal prep not only empowers you to make healthier choices over the tempting vending machine, but it also ensures that you stay energized and focused, ready to tackle whatever challenges come your way during those demanding hours on the job.

Now, let's dive into the topic of budget. As a busy nurse or dedicated nursing student, you're likely balancing your finances as skillfully as you manage patient charts. The good news is that eating healthy doesn't have to drain your wallet or cost an arm and a leg. Picture this: you can create an entire week's worth of delicious, nutritious meals using the same budget you typically allocate to your daily fancy coffee habit. By embracing meal prep, you can tap into your inner chef without needing to perform financial acrobatics. You'll soon discover that by buying in bulk and incorporating budget-friendly ingredients, you can transform yourself into a culinary genius—no culinary school required and no gourmet experience necessary.

For those night shifts where you feel like a zombie in scrubs, high-energy snacks truly become your best friends. Instead of reaching for yet another sugary snack that inevitably leads to a frustrating crash, taking the time to meal prep allows you to whip up delicious, protein-packed snacks that effectively keep you alert and focused throughout your shift. Consider making homemade energy balls or assembling veggie cups filled with creamy hummus, all ready to go whenever you need a much-needed pick-me-up. You'll not only feel significantly better and more energized, but your colleagues might even become curious and ask for your secret recipe—what a fantastic way to bond over something other than caffeine and share healthy eating habits!

So, why should you consider trading in your morning coffee IV for a comprehensive meal prep plan? While caffeine might provide you with a fleeting boost of energy, meal prepping offers you the tools to maintain stable energy levels and promote overall wellness throughout your busy days. You truly deserve to nourish your body with wholesome, nutritious foods that align with your demanding lifestyle and help you thrive. With a bit of thoughtful planning and a sprinkle of creativity, you can tackle those long shifts, delight your taste buds with delicious meals, and potentially save some money in the process. After all, nursing is undeniably challenging; you shouldn't have to struggle with hunger and fatigue while navigating your responsibilities.

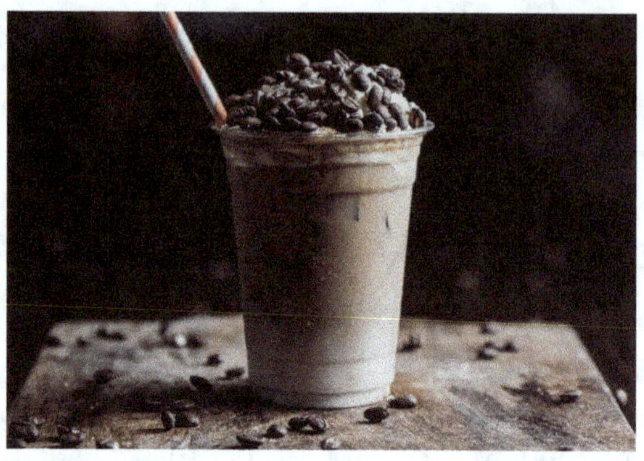

Time Management: Don't Let Your Dinner Shift Play the First Shift

Time management in the life of a nurse is akin to juggling flaming torches while riding a unicycle on a tightrope high above the ground. With shifts that can stretch into the twilight hours and a schedule that shifts more than a toddler at bedtime, it's absolutely crucial to ensure that your dinner doesn't decide to play the first shift instead of you. After all, no one wants to be the nurse who survives on vending machine snacks, stale granola bars, and cold pizza that has been sitting out for hours, right? Let's dive into some hilariously practical tips and clever strategies to keep your meal prep game strong while you navigate the delightful chaos of your nursing career, ensuring that you stay nourished and energized throughout those demanding shifts.

Time management in the life of a nurse is akin to juggling flaming torches while riding a unicycle on a tightrope high above the ground. With shifts that can stretch into the twilight hours and a schedule that shifts more than a toddler at bedtime, it's absolutely crucial to ensure that your dinner doesn't decide to play the first shift instead of you. After all, no one wants to be the nurse who survives on vending machine snacks, stale granola bars, and cold pizza that has been sitting out for hours, right? Let's dive into some hilariously practical tips and clever strategies to keep your meal prep game strong while you navigate the delightful chaos of your nursing career, ensuring that you stay nourished and energized throughout those demanding shifts.

First off, let's dive into the essential topic of meal prep. You might think it's just for Instagram influencers and those mythical creatures known as "stay-at-home parents," but let me tell you, for us nurses, it's an absolute necessity. Imagine this scenario: you come home after a grueling 12-hour shift, and the last thing you want to do is wrestle with a can of beans and a box of something suspicious that you unearthed from the back of your pantry. Instead, dedicate a Sunday to channel your inner chef, or at least your inner "I can microwave this in under two minutes." Chop, sauté, and pack your meals with the same enthusiasm as if you're prepping for a high-stakes reality cooking show. Trust me, when you find yourself exhausted and the only thing standing between you and a hot, satisfying meal is a quick trip to the fridge, you'll be grateful for the effort you put in ahead of time. This simple act of preparation can transform your week and save you from the stress of last-minute cooking.

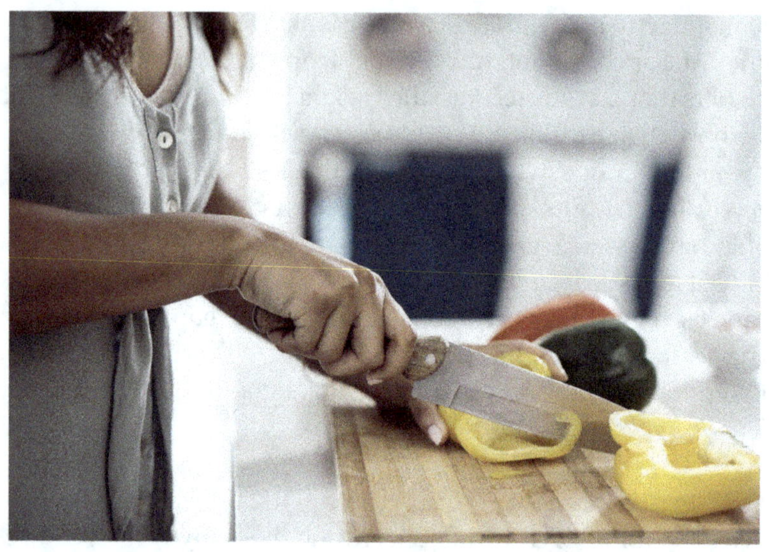

Now, let's not forget about those quick and easy recipes that require little more than a microwave and a dash of culinary courage. Think about meals that yell "I'm healthy and I won't devour all your precious time." How about a five-minute omelet? Yes, please! What about a vibrant salad that doesn't require a degree in agriculture or a lifetime of gardening experience? Sign me up! The key here is to wholeheartedly embrace simplicity while adding a sprinkle of creativity. Just toss some leftover chicken, a handful of fresh greens, and your favorite dressing in a bowl, and voila! You've just created a culinary masterpiece that even Picasso would envy, assuming he was both hungry and possessed a solid understanding of nutrition and flavor balance. So, don't hesitate to experiment and enjoy the process!

For the nursing students out there, low-budget meals can feel like the holy grail of culinary art, a treasure trove of delicious possibilities without the hefty price tag. You don't need to break the bank to eat well and nourish your body. Think ramen, but not the kind that comes with a side of regret or disappointment. By adding some frozen veggies and a perfectly cooked egg, you can transform that humble dish into a delightful feast that makes you feel like royalty while living the student life. It's all about the clever hacks and resourcefulness, my friends. Canned beans, hearty rice, and a dash of hot sauce can be combined to create a meal that will fuel you through the next demanding clinical shift without requiring you to take out a second mortgage. Embrace these budget-friendly strategies, and you'll find that eating well is both achievable and enjoyable.

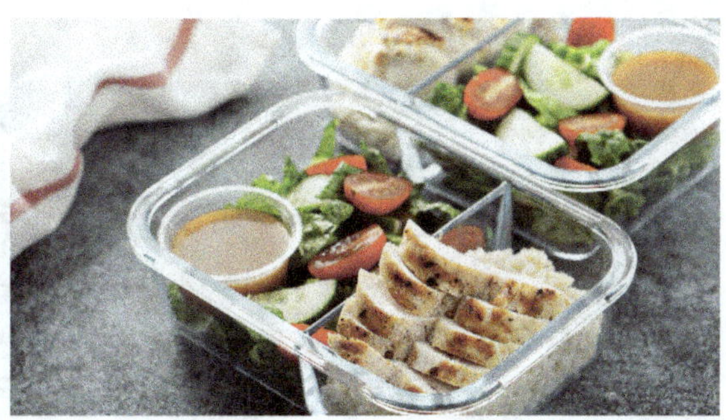

Finally, let's dive into the topic of snacks because, let's face it, trying to survive those long shifts on caffeine alone is a guaranteed recipe for disaster. High-energy snacks are truly your best friends in this demanding environment, and they shouldn't merely consist of a sad collection of granola bars that you find crumpled at the bottom of your bag. Instead, consider whipping up your own energy bites using wholesome oats, creamy peanut butter, and a delightful sprinkle of chocolate chips—because really, who doesn't deserve a touch of sweetness to brighten up a grueling night? Pack these tasty treats in your scrubs pocket, and you'll have a delicious pick-me-up ready to go when those inevitable 3 a.m. hunger pangs strike. Keep in mind that the key to thriving in the nursing world lies in managing your time wisely, so while you're busy saving lives, your dinner can rest easy— and maybe, just maybe, you'll get to enjoy a few snacks along the way.

Kitchen Gadgets: Your New Best Friends (Sorry, Stethoscope

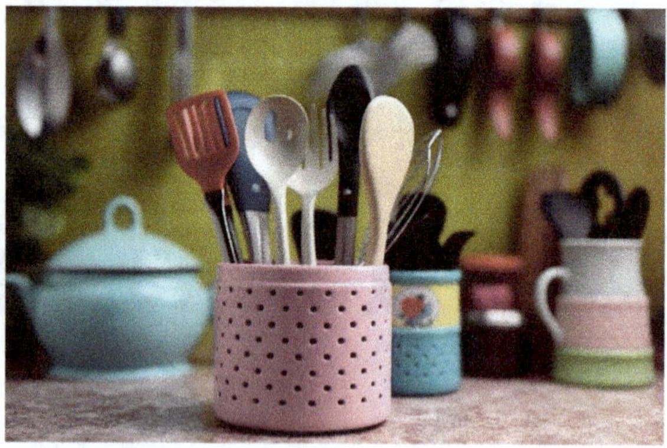

When you're a busy nurse juggling demanding shifts and a hectic schedule, meal prep might seem like an indulgence reserved only for those fortunate enough to have the luxury of time to binge-watch cooking shows or experiment in the kitchen. But fear not, fellow nurses! Innovative kitchen gadgets are here to rescue you from the tyranny of takeout menus and the ever-haunting echoes of "What's for dinner?" that can often plague our evenings after long, exhausting days. With the right tools at your disposal, you can whip up delicious and nutritious meals faster than you can say, "Sorry, I can't talk right now; I'm on a break!" Embrace these time-saving devices and reclaim your evenings, transforming them into a time for enjoying wholesome, home-cooked meals that nourish your body and soul. You deserve to savor the fruits of your labor in the comfort of your own kitchen, all while keeping your energy up for the demanding work you do.

First up on our gadget hit parade is the ever-reliable Instant Pot. This remarkable multi-cooker is like the superhero of the kitchen—faster than a speeding bullet, capable of tenderizing even the toughest cuts of meat in a single bound, and absolutely perfect for crafting delicious soups, hearty stews, and even creamy yogurt (because you never know when that unexpected midnight yogurt craving might strike). Just toss in your carefully selected ingredients, set the timer, and while the Instant Pot works its culinary magic, you can take a well-deserved breather or even perfect your power pose for the next shift ahead. Sure, it might not have the same ring or prestige as "stethoscope," but it will undoubtedly earn a cherished spot in your heart and kitchen routine.

Next, let's delve into the air fryer, a kitchen appliance that has truly taken the culinary world by storm and revolutionized the way we prepare our favorite foods. It's the guilt-free way to indulge in crispy snacks without the need for a traditional deep fryer and an excessive amount of oil. Picture this: perfectly crispy sweet potato fries or delightfully crunchy chickpeas, all while effortlessly maintaining your healthy eating goals and lifestyle. Additionally, it's the perfect gadget for those late-night cravings when you find yourself needing something quick, delicious, and satisfying between shifts. Just don't be surprised if you start dreaming about your air fryer; it's a love affair with convenience and flavor that's incredibly hard to resist!

For those of you who prefer the "set it and forget it" approach to cooking, a slow cooker might just become your new best friend and kitchen companion. You can easily prepare a hearty chili or a nutritious stew before your shift begins, and by the time you return home, your meal will be hot, flavorful, and ready to eat without any additional effort. It's almost like having a personal chef who never complains about the long hours or asks for time off. Just remember to set an alarm or timer, so you don't end up with a science experiment gone wrong instead of a delicious dinner—you know, the kind that makes you seriously question your life choices and culinary skills.

Finally, let's take a moment to give a well-deserved shout-out to the blender. This little dynamo is truly perfect for whipping up smoothies loaded with energy-boosting ingredients that will help you power through those long and demanding shifts. Just toss in some vibrant spinach, an assortment of frozen fruits, and a generous scoop of protein powder, and you've effortlessly created a quick meal that's both nutritious and absolutely delicious. Plus, using a blender makes you feel like a culinary genius, effortlessly blending everything together in mere seconds. Just remember to clean it right away; nobody wants to return home after a long shift only to confront the horror of a crusty, unwashed blender staring back at them.

So, as you navigate through the demands of your busy nursing life, always keep in mind that kitchen gadgets can be invaluable allies in your quest for healthy, quick, and budget-friendly meals. While they may not possess the same elegance or flair as your trusted stethoscope, these handy gadgets certainly excel at helping you stay nourished and flourishing, one nutritious meal at a time! Embracing their convenience can make a significant difference in maintaining your well-being amidst your hectic schedule.

02 Quick and Easy Recipes for Night Shifts

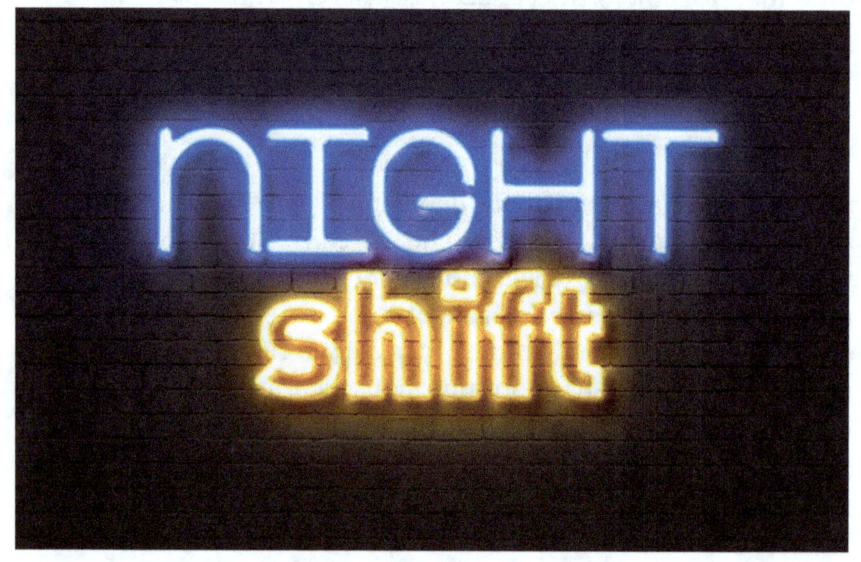

Breakfast for Dinner: Because Who Says Eggs Can't Fly at Midnight?

Breakfast for dinner is the culinary equivalent of wearing pajamas to the grocery store—delightfully rebellious and deliciously comforting. For nurses who have spent their day (or night) saving lives, the thought of whipping up a gourmet meal feels as daunting as trying to teach a cat to fetch or trying to solve a complicated puzzle after a long shift. Enter the enchanting world of breakfast for dinner, where eggs can be scrambled at any hour, and pancakes are just as acceptable at midnight as they are at dawn. It's the culinary freedom every busy nurse desperately needs, especially after a long, exhausting shift when all you want is something quick, easy, and utterly satisfying. Imagine indulging in a stack of fluffy pancakes topped with syrup or diving into a warm bowl of oatmeal, knowing that the comfort of breakfast is just a few moments away.

Eggs are the superheroes of the breakfast-for-dinner world, effortlessly bridging the gap between breakfast and dinner with their versatility. Packed with protein, they can easily transform from a morning staple to a midnight feast that satisfies your hunger. Simply throw them into a frittata along with whatever leftover veggies are lurking in your fridge, and voilà, you've got a meal that's not only quick to prepare but also a vibrant and colorful display of culinary creativity. Plus, let's not forget that they cook faster than a student

cramming for finals, making them the perfect choice for those who
are short on time. In just a matter of minutes, you can have a plateful
of fluffy goodness that fuels you for those late-night charting
sessions and keeps your energy levels up while you tackle your
workload.

.

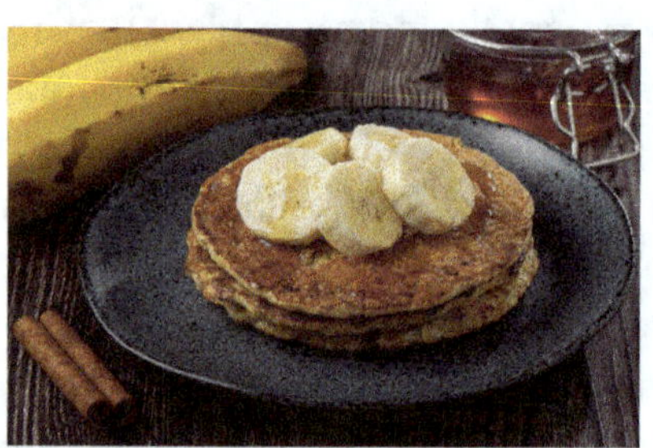

But what about those who prefer a touch of sweetness in their
meals? Enter pancakes, those delightful, magical discs of joy that
can be adorned with an endless array of toppings, ranging from rich
syrup to creamy peanut butter, and even the last bit of fruit before it
reaches its expiration. A pancake dinner is not only a delightful and
whimsical deviation from the everyday norm but also an
opportunity to unleash your inner artist. You can create pancake
faces that would make even Picasso stand in awe, all while relishing
the satisfaction that comes from transforming a breakfast favorite
into a nutritional powerhouse. Who would have thought that a
simple stack of pancakes could ignite so much joy and happiness at
the stroke of midnight?

For nurses on a budget, breakfast for dinner can truly be an economical delight that satisfies both taste and financial constraints. A dozen eggs and a bag of flour can stretch further than a pair of compression socks on a grueling long shift. When you add in some seasonal fruits or veggies, you'll find you have a variety of meals that won't break the bank, allowing you to enjoy delicious, nutritious options without overspending. Plus, don't forget about the communal break room; you can always raid it for those leftover muffins or granola bars that your coworkers are undoubtedly hoarding. Think of it as your late-night scavenger hunt—who knew you could discover inspiration for a satisfying dinner in a box of stale doughnuts? Embrace the challenge and turn simple ingredients and communal treasures into a delightful feast!

Finally, let's not forget the importance of snacks during those long shifts. High-energy snacks can truly be the lifeblood of a nurse's night shift, and there's really no better way to fuel up than with delicious breakfast-inspired treats that are both satisfying and nourishing. Overnight oats can be a healthy, easy-to-prep snack that you can conveniently grab on the go when time is tight, or why not whip up some energy balls packed with a variety of nuts and seeds? These little power-packed bites are the perfect midnight pick-me-up when you need a little boost to keep you going through those endless and demanding shifts.

So, don't shy away from the comforting breakfast foods that can easily fly at midnight; embrace them fully, and you'll discover that breakfast for dinner is not just a simple meal choice, but a vibrant lifestyle that nourishes and flourishes in the busy lives of nurses everywhere, making those challenging nights just a bit more enjoyable.

One-Pan Wonders: Less Cleaning, More Napping

After an exhausting 12-hour shift where your hands have been busier than a one-armed wallpaper hanger, the absolute last thing you want to do is transform into a culinary Picasso in the kitchen. Enter the enchanting realm of one-pan wonders, where all that is required of you is to master the fine art of not burning the house down in the process. These delightful recipes not only promise a feast for your taste buds but also ensure that your well-deserved post-shift downtime is spent blissfully napping rather than frantically scrubbing pots and pans like a character trapped in a kitchen horror movie. With these easy-to-follow meals, you can enjoy delicious flavors without the hassle of extensive cleanup, allowing you to truly relax and recharge.'

Picture this: you stumble into your kitchen, hair a disheveled mess and feet aching as if you've just completed a grueling marathon. You open the fridge, and instead of being greeted by a daunting array of ingredients that demand a Michelin star-level of finesse, you find a handful of colorful veggies, some tender chicken, and a rogue jar of zesty salsa hiding in the back. With just one trusty pan and a sprinkle of unshakeable optimism, you can toss everything together and let the oven do the heavy lifting for you. Before you know it, you'll have a delicious and satisfying meal that requires minimal effort and absolutely zero culinary training. It's a culinary miracle! Bonus points if you can pull this off while still comfortably wearing your scrubs, proving that you can conquer the kitchen in style, no matter how hectic your day has been!

'Now, let's dive into the beauty of low-budget meals, which truly are a nurse's best friend—because let's face it, our student loans are probably still haunting us like a ghost in a classic horror film that just won't let go. One-pan meals are absolutely perfect for utilizing those random leftovers and that sad-looking produce lurking at the back of the fridge, waiting for a chance to shine. You can easily throw together a delicious stir-fry using yesterday's rice and whatever vegetables are practically begging for rescue from their unfortunate fate. Just think of it as your fridge's last-ditch effort to avoid becoming a compost pile, fighting to stay relevant in your culinary adventures. And the absolute best part? You'll save enough money to treat yourself to some well-deserved takeout after your next long shift, allowing you to indulge a little without the guilt!

And speaking of energy, we all know how incredibly important it is to maintain high spirits during those long, exhausting shifts that can really take a toll on our well-being. One-pan wonders can be easily modified into high-energy snacks that will have you feeling like a superhero instead of a sleep-deprived zombie struggling to get through the day. Imagine indulging in delicious roasted chickpeas or perfectly spiced nuts, both of which can be made in bulk and stored conveniently for those moments when you desperately need something quick, nutritious, and satisfying. With just a single baking sheet, you can whip up a delightful variety of snacks that not only fuel your body but also keep your energy levels elevated enough to tackle those demanding night shifts without the constant risk of dozing off on the job. These simple yet effective snack options serve as a fantastic solution to ensure you remain alert and energized throughout those long hours, making the experience much more manageable and enjoyable.

So, gather your favorite one-pan recipes and let them serve as your culinary lifeline in the whirlwind of your busy life. Embrace the simplicity and ease that come with cooking in just one vessel, allowing yourself the precious gift of time that you can use to nap, binge-watch the latest episodes of your favorite show, or even finally dive into that book that's been collecting dust on your nightstand for far too long. After all, life as a nurse can be wonderfully chaotic, but your meals don't have to follow suit. With a healthy dash of creativity and a sprinkle of humor, you'll be well-equipped to nourish your body, thrive in your role, and enjoy those moments of relaxation—all while skillfully dodging the dreaded post-dinner dishwashing marathon that often seems to linger on the horizon.

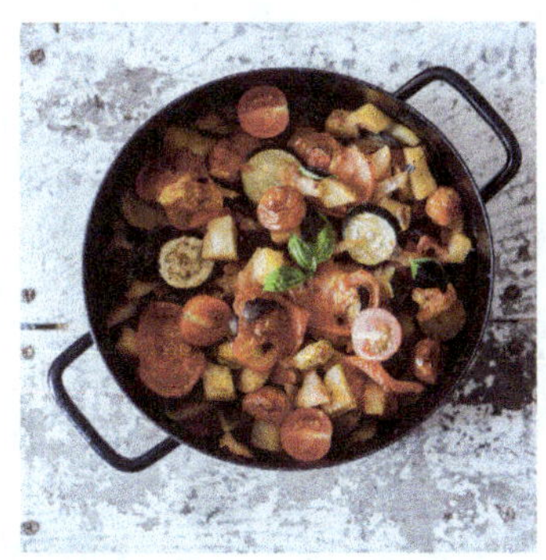

Freezer-Friendly Favorites: Prepare, Freeze, and Forget (Until You're Starving!)

Freezer-friendly meals are like your favorite pair of scrubs: reliable, comfortable, and always there when you need them most. After a long shift at the hospital, the last thing you want to do is spend an hour in the kitchen preparing dinner. Instead, imagine the relief of opening your freezer and being greeted by a delicious, nutritious meal, just waiting for you like a loyal puppy eager for a walk in the park. The beauty of freezer-friendly meals is that with a little prep work on your day off, you can ensure that you never have to face the dreaded 'what's for dinner?' dilemma again. This means you can spend significantly less time cooking and more time indulging in binge-watching your favorite medical dramas or catching up on those captivating soap operas, because let's face it, even dedicated nurses deserve their moments of relaxation and entertainment.

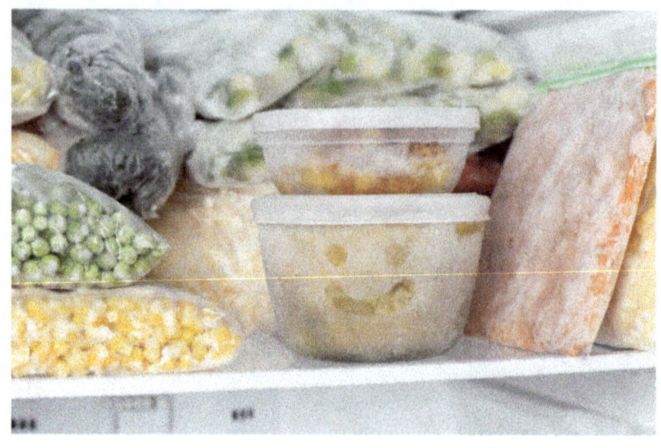

First up on the freezer-friendly favorites list is the classic chili, a timeless favorite loved by many. You can prepare a massive pot of it in less time than it takes to complete a medication round, making it a perfect choice for busy schedules. Load it with plenty of beans, colorful veggies, and lean meats, allowing it to simmer gently like a soothing cup of tea, filling your kitchen with delightful aromas. Once it cools down, ladle it into freezer bags—just don't forget to label them! "Chili" is much more appetizing than the ambiguous "mystery meal." When those hunger pangs hit after a long night shift, you can simply thaw it out, heat it up, and enjoy a bowl of warmth that rivals the comfort of your favorite blanket. Pro tip: keep a stash of cornbread mix on hand for those nights when you want to elevate your meal from a simple "nurse's dinner" to a "gourmet restaurant experience" that will impress even the most discerning palate.

Next, let's dive deeper into the world of stir-fries. They're the true superheroes of freezer meals, swooping in to rescue you from potential kitchen disasters when time is short and hunger strikes. You can chop up any delightful combination of colorful vegetables, various proteins, and flavorful sauces, toss them all in a sizzling pan, and voilà! Portion out your delicious creations into freezer-safe containers, and you've got a meal that's as versatile and adaptable as your trusty stethoscope. Craving a savory beef stir-fry one night and a refreshing tofu version the next? No problem at all! Just grab a container from your freezer, toss it in the microwave, and in no time at all, you're ready to enjoy a tasty meal faster than you can say "I'll take the night shift."

For those shifts when you find yourself in need of a snack that truly packs a punch, consider freezing some delicious energy balls. These little bites of joy are not only satisfying but can also be easily made from a base of oats, nut butter, and any other ingredients you happen to have lying around, such as chocolate chips, dried fruit, or even seeds. Simply roll them into bite-sized balls, pop them in

the freezer, and you'll have a convenient stash of high-energy snacks ready to keep you fueled through those long night shifts. Plus, they're incredibly easy to grab and go, making them perfect for those busy moments when you're rushing from one patient to the next. Just be prepared for your coworkers to start asking you for your secret recipe—you might find yourself needing to start a snack club to share the joy!

Finally, let's not forget about soups. They are the ultimate comfort food, especially on those days when you're running on little sleep and even less patience. Whip up a big batch of your favorite soup, whether it's a hearty minestrone packed with vegetables and beans or a creamy butternut squash that warms you from the inside out. Portion it out into freezer-friendly containers, and you'll always have a delicious bowl of goodness waiting for you, ready to be enjoyed at a moment's notice. The best part? You can savor it while wearing your favorite pajamas because, honestly, who has the energy to get dressed after a grueling 12-hour shift? So go ahead, prepare, freeze, and forget about it—until you're starving, of course! And when that hunger pangs hit, you'll be grateful you took the time to stock your freezer with such a comforting meal!

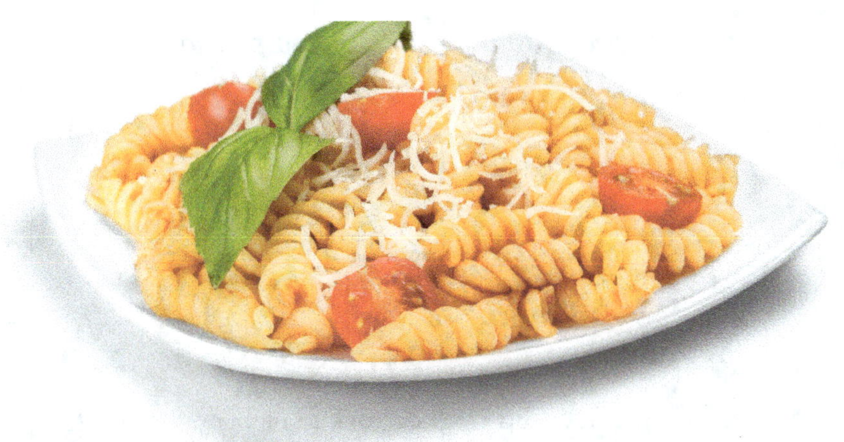

03

Low-Budget Meals for Nursing Students

Ramen Reinvented: From Instant to Incredible!

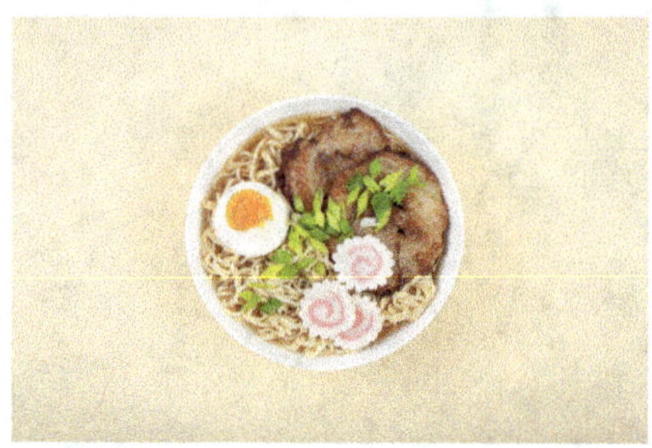

Ramen has long been the unsung hero of late-night nursing shifts, often regarded as the culinary equivalent of a trusty old stethoscope that never lets you down. You know the drill: you're knee-deep in paperwork, the clock is ticking, and the only thing standing between you and a full-blown meltdown is that comforting little cup of instant ramen. But let's be real—while it's convenient and quick, it's not exactly a dish worthy of a Michelin star. So, how do we elevate this humble noodle bowl from a sad desk lunch to something truly exceptional that'll have you feeling like a culinary rock star? Welcome to the exciting world of "Ramen Reinvented: From Instant to Incredible," where we explore ways to transform this simple meal into a gourmet experience.

First, let's dive into the basics of ramen. While it may often be viewed as a quick and convenient fix for hunger, it doesn't have to be a nutritional black hole that leaves you feeling empty. By simply ditching that flavor packet, which is more about salt than actual spice, and adding your own personal touch (along with some essential nutrients!), you can completely transform your instant ramen into a truly wholesome meal. Imagine it as the noodle version of a superhero, ready to save the day. Toss in an array of sautéed vegetables—think spinach, bell peppers, or whatever treasures you can find lurking in your fridge that won't put up a fight—and you've got yourself a vibrant, vitamin-packed dish that's bursting with color and flavor. It's like giving your ramen a much-needed spa day, revitalizing it into something delightful and nourishing.

Now, let's not forget about the importance of protein. We really need to fuel those long shifts, right? Instead of leaving your ramen to fend for itself in a sea of carbs, why not consider adding an egg? Cracking a soft-boiled egg on top of your steaming noodles is like putting a crown on your ramen—instant royalty and a delightful touch! But hey, if you're feeling a bit fancy (and have a little time to spare), try poaching that egg directly in the broth. Just imagine how impressed you'll be as the egg swirls in the warm liquid, creating a beautiful blend of flavors. You'll be the envy of your fellow nurses as you casually slurp your elevated bowl of noodles, all while they're still trying to figure out how to open that cup of instant. They'll be wondering how you've mastered such a delicious upgrade!

For those adventurous souls among you, let's really spice things up —literally speaking. A little bit of heat can go an incredibly long way in transforming your ramen experience into something truly extraordinary and memorable. A simple dash of sriracha or a generous sprinkle of chili flakes can awaken even the sleepiest of taste buds, making every single bite an exciting journey filled with flavor. If you're feeling particularly daring and bold, you could even

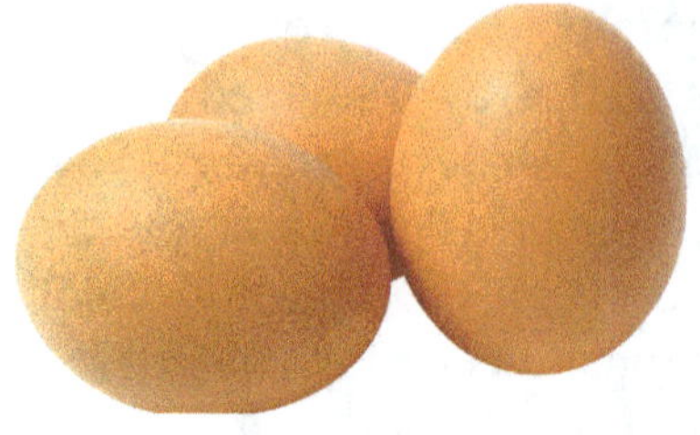

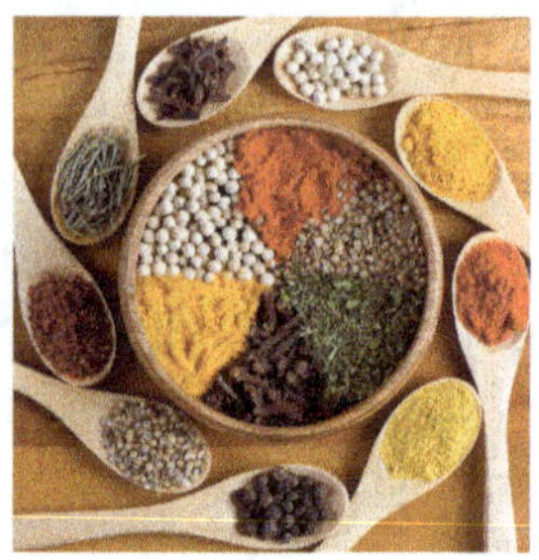

take it a step further by crafting a homemade broth infused with aromatic ginger, savory garlic, and perhaps a hint of fresh lime for that extra zing. Just imagine the delightful aroma wafting through the break room—your co-workers will undoubtedly think you've just returned from an exotic culinary retreat instead of enduring a grueling 12-hour shift. They might even be tempted to ask for a taste of your delicious creation, turning an ordinary meal into a delightful sharing experience.

Finally, let's dive into the topic of budget. We all know that nursing school can leave your wallet feeling like it's on a strict diet, and managing finances can be quite a challenge. Fortunately, ramen has long been recognized as the ultimate poster child for low-budget meals that are both satisfying and versatile. By investing in a few essential staple ingredients like frozen veggies, eggs, and perhaps some lean protein, you can whip up a week's worth of delicious, nutritious meals without breaking the bank or sacrificing flavor. Moreover, meal prepping a batch of ramen bowls means you can conveniently grab and go during those chaotic shifts, ensuring you stay nourished and energized throughout your demanding days. So go ahead, embrace the ramen renaissance—because even the most dedicated superheroes need a delicious meal to fuel their efforts and save the day!

Pantry Staples: The Superheroes of Your Kitchen

Pantry staples are like the unsung heroes of your kitchen, quietly waiting on the shelves while you dash around in a whirlwind of scrubs and caffeine, often overlooked but always ready to support you. These trusty ingredients form the essential foundation of your culinary adventures, poised to spring into action when hunger strikes unexpectedly in the middle of a grueling 12-hour shift. You might believe that crafting a delicious and satisfying meal requires an elaborate gourmet grocery list, but the reality is that your pantry is likely bursting with untapped potential just waiting to be explored. With a little creativity and imagination, those humble cans of beans and bags of rice can easily transform into a feast fit for a superhero —or at least something far more exciting and satisfying than yet another bland microwaved meal. Embracing these pantry staples can lead to surprising culinary delights that not only nourish your body but also invigorate your spirit after a long day.

First up in our pantry superhero lineup is the mighty can of beans. These little legumes, bursting with goodness, are packed with protein and fiber, making them the perfect sidekick for any meal you can imagine. Toss them into a vibrant salad, blend them into a creamy dip, or throw them into a hearty burrito bowl for a quick and satisfying dinner that will leave you feeling full and energized. And let's not forget how they can save you from the dreaded "I forgot to eat" moment during your long night shift. Just picture this: you're in the break room, desperately searching for food to fuel your work, and there they are, your trusty beans, ready to save the day and keep you going strong. Plus, they're incredibly budget-friendly, so you can save your hard-earned cash for more important things—like that essential cup of coffee that keeps you alert and focused.

Next, we have rice, the incredibly versatile sidekick that every busy nurse should always have on hand in their kitchen. Whether you prefer the wholesome texture of brown rice, the classic appeal of white rice, or even the trendy cauliflower rice, this carbohydrate champion can serve as the foundation for countless delicious meals. Feeling adventurous? Why not make a stir-fry using whatever fresh veggies you can find in the fridge, or whip up a hearty one-pot dish with tender chicken and a flavorful blend of spices that will truly make your taste buds dance with delight. And if you're really pressed for time during those long shifts, you can always prepare a generous batch of rice over the weekend and simply reheat it on those hectic night shifts. It's like having a reliable culinary sidekick that's always there for you, even when you're running low on energy and just need a quick, satisfying meal to keep you going.

Don't overlook the incredible power of pasta, either! This beloved culinary staple has the amazing ability to transform a pile of random ingredients into a comforting and satisfying meal faster than you can say "carb-loading." Spaghetti tossed with canned tomatoes and minced garlic? Instant classic that never disappoints. Mac and cheese made from whatever cheese you have stashed in your pantry? Yes, please! Plus, pasta possesses the uncanny ability

to elevate your cooking experience, making you feel like a gourmet chef without the fuss and intimidation often associated with fine dining. A sprinkle of fresh herbs here, a generous dash of high-quality olive oil there, and suddenly you're presenting a dish that would make even Gordon Ramsay nod in approval—though, to be fair, he might still find a reason to yell at you for not using fresh ingredients or for some other minor infraction.

Let's not forget the incredible magic of spices, the true superheroes of the culinary world that pack a powerful punch in flavor while taking up minimal space in your kitchen. Just a little sprinkle of cumin, a dash of chili powder, or a spoonful of garlic powder can effortlessly elevate your pantry staples from dull and bland to grand and exciting in mere seconds. It's almost like giving your meals a superhero cape, allowing them to soar off the plate and delightfully into your mouth. With a well-stocked spice rack at your fingertips, you can transform a simple can of tomatoes into a vibrant, zesty salsa or make those humble beans sing with an explosion of flavor. So go ahead, sprinkle that magic dust on your meals and let your taste buds take an exhilarating flight into a world of deliciousness.

Finally, we must take a moment to salute the healthy snacks that truly deserve a prominent place in your pantry. Nuts, dried fruits, and whole-grain crackers are not just tasty but are also the perfect fuel to keep you energized and focused during those long, demanding shifts. They're portable, incredibly easy to munch on, and best of all, they don't require a microwave or any fancy preparation. When the clock strikes snack-o'clock, you'll be exceptionally glad you have a stash of these nutritious goodies to keep you going strong. Just remember to conceal them from your curious colleagues unless you're fully prepared to share the delightful secret of your superhero snack stash. With these essential pantry staples by your side, you'll be more than ready to conquer your shifts, one delicious and satisfying meal at a time!

Meal Prep on a Dime: How to Eat Well Without Selling Your Soul

Meal prep can sometimes feel like an unattainable luxury, reserved only for those fortunate enough to have endless funds and an entire arsenal of high-end kitchen gadgets. But fear not, busy nurses! You definitely don't need to part with your soul (or even your kidney) just to enjoy nutritious meals that nourish both your body and spirit. With a dash of creativity, a pinch of resourcefulness, and a generous sprinkle of humor, you can easily whip up a variety of delicious, nutritious meals that won't drain your wallet or dampen your enthusiasm. Think of it as a thrilling game show challenge where the ultimate prize is not just maintaining your sanity, but also enhancing your health and overall well-being—no pressure, right? Embrace this culinary adventure, savor the process, and enjoy every delightful moment along the way.

First things first, let's dive into the art of shopping smart. Channel your inner bargain hunter as you skillfully navigate the grocery store. You know the aisles like the back of your hand, so make a beeline for the sales and discounts. Don't forget to stock up on seasonal fruits and veggies—they're not only cheaper and fresher, but they also give you that magical glow that proudly says, "I'm a responsible adult who knows how to shop wisely!" And while you're at it, don't overlook those canned and frozen options; they're often just as nutritious and way less pricey than their fresh counterparts. Just be sure to check the labels carefully—no one needs a surprise ingredient list that reads like a horror novel filled with unrecognizable additives and preservatives. Shopping smart is all about making informed choices that benefit your wallet and your well-being.

Now that you're loaded up with a fantastic selection of affordable goodies, it's time to dive into the wonderful world of cooking. Meal prep doesn't have to mean slaving away over the stove like a contestant on a high-pressure cooking show. Instead, grab your trusty slow cooker or Instant Pot and let it do all the heavy lifting while you comfortably settle in and binge-watch your favorite medical drama or any show that captivates you. Just toss in some beans, rice, and those vegetables that are nearing their last legs in your fridge, and let that cooking magic happen. Before you know it, you'll have a week's worth of delicious meals that taste like you've been slaving away for hours in the kitchen, when in reality, you were simply enjoying your best couch potato life, effortlessly combining relaxation with smart meal planning.

Let's not forget about snacks—those essential little energy boosts that keep you going strong during those long, demanding shifts. Say goodbye to the vending machine and hello to delicious, homemade high-energy snacks that are as easy as pie (but we promise they're much healthier). Imagine creating your own trail mix, packed with a delightful combination of nuts, seeds, and a few chocolate chips for that perfect touch of sweetness. Or consider whipping up some tasty energy balls using wholesome oats, creamy nut butter, and a drizzle of honey. These delightful little bites will not only keep you fueled but also make you feel like a superhero, ready to tackle whatever challenges the night shift throws your way. Plus, they're significantly cheaper than those overpriced granola bars that often taste like cardboard, allowing you to snack smarter without breaking the bank.

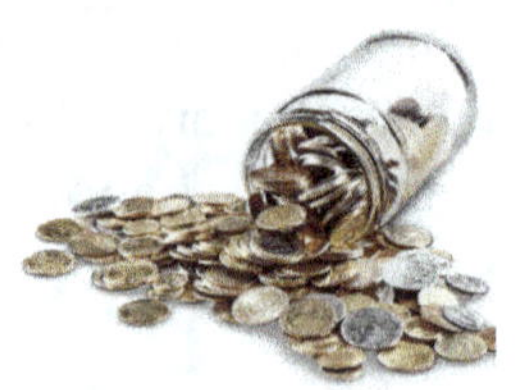

Finally, let's address the all-too-common "I don't have time" excuse. Seriously, who actually has time these days? You're a dedicated nurse, after all! But here's the important thing to consider: meal prep can genuinely save you a significant amount of time in the long run, much more than you might realize. Imagine this scenario: if you set aside just a couple of hours on your day off, you could cook and portion out your meals for the week ahead. Picture how much you'll be thanking yourself later for this small investment of time. No more frantic searches for something to eat in the break room or settling for unhealthy snacks that leave you feeling sluggish. Instead, you'll have an array of nutritious options right at your fingertips, ready to go before you even have to take off your scrubs after a long shift. So, grab those trusty Tupperware containers, put on some music, and let's redefine what it truly means to eat well on a budget. You've absolutely got this, and your body will thank you for making these smart choices!

04

High-Energy Snacks for Long Shifts

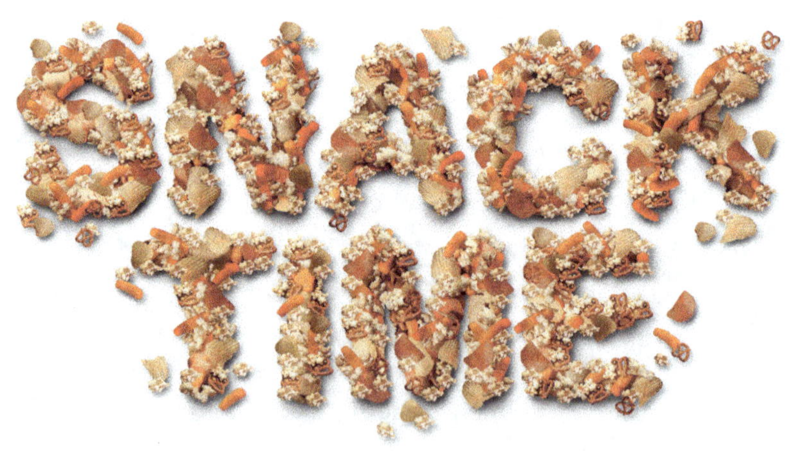

Snack Attack: Things to Munch That Won't Make You Crash

Let's face it, nurses are undoubtedly the superheroes of the medical world, but even the most dedicated superheroes need to take a moment to refuel. When the clock's hands are spinning like the wheel of fortune, and you're fighting off the overwhelming urge to nap on your feet, the very last thing you want is for your snack to transform into a villain in your day. We're talking about those sugary treats that might give you a quick rush of energy, only to leave you crashing harder than a patient's blood pressure after too much salt. Instead of falling into that trap, let's take a moment to explore some nutritious snack options that will help keep your energy levels steady and your spirits high, all without the dramatic plot twists that can derail your focus and productivity.

First on the list is the mighty nut butter. Whether it's almond, peanut, or even that trendy sunflower seed butter that's been gaining popularity, these little jars of joy are packed with healthy fats and protein that can fuel your day. Grab a generous spoonful or spread it luxuriously on whole-grain toast, and you've got yourself a delightful snack that won't send you spiraling into a sugar coma or leaving you feeling sluggish afterward. Plus, they're incredibly portable! So, when you find yourself in the break room, armed with only your trusty snack stash, you can confidently whip out your nut butter without fear of judgment from your colleagues. Just make sure to bring some crisp apple slices or whole-grain crackers along; otherwise, you might as well be eating it straight from the jar like a true snack-time rebel, indulging in that creamy goodness without a care in the world.

Next up, we have the often underappreciated hero of healthy snacking: Greek yogurt. It's creamy, it's dreamy, and it's absolutely loaded with protein to keep you feeling full and satisfied during those long, demanding shifts. Toss in some fresh berries or a generous sprinkle of granola, and you've got yourself a delightful snack that even the pickiest of taste buds will applaud and appreciate. And let's not forget about the amazing probiotics—your gut will be dancing with joy like it just won the lottery and received a surprise vacation. Just be careful with the flavored varieties; while a little sugar is perfectly fine, you definitely don't want to end up with a yogurt that contains more sweetness than a candy bar. We're aiming for sustained energy, not a sugar rush that leaves you face-down and exhausted in the nursing station, struggling to stay awake.

Now, if you're on the hunt for a snack that feels indulgent yet won't leave you second-guessing your life choices, look no further than popcorn. Yes, that delightful fluffy goodness can transform into a guilt-free pleasure if you keep it uncomplicated. Ditch the butter and heavy toppings, and instead, go for air-popped popcorn seasoned with just a pinch of salt or some nutritional yeast for an extra flavor boost. It's light, crunchy, and will keep your hands occupied during those slow moments when you're desperately trying to stay awake. Plus, it's so budget-friendly that you'll still have plenty of cash left over to treat yourself to that fancy coffee you've been craving. Just be ready for the occasional rogue kernel that decides to jump ship; it's basically the popcorn equivalent of a nursing student forgetting their stethoscope, adding a little unpredictability to your snacking experience.

Lastly, let's not overlook the incredible power of the humble energy ball. These bite-sized snacks are like little nuggets of pure joy that can be whipped up in no time at all. Simply combine oats, nut butter, honey, and then toss in some chocolate chips or dried fruit, and voilà! You've got a delightful snack that's as easy to make as it is to eat. Plus, they're absolutely perfect for stashing in your scrubs or bag, ready to be devoured during those chaotic moments when the coffee line is infinitely longer than the patient queue. Just remember to keep them in a container unless you want your bag to resemble a granola explosion, which can be quite the mess. With these tasty snacks in your arsenal, you'll be able to conquer your shift like the superhero you truly are—one satisfying munch at a time, ensuring you have the energy to tackle whatever comes your way.

DIY Energy Bites: No More Expensive Store-Bought Lies

DIY energy bites are the superhero snacks we never knew we needed and have been missing out on for far too long. Forget those overpriced, store-bought lies that promise energy and health benefits but leave your wallet feeling as light as your eyelids after a long, exhausting shift. These little power balls are not only budget-friendly but also incredibly quick and easy to whip up, making them the perfect sidekick for busy nurses who desperately need a boost during those grueling, marathon shifts. Why settle for a snack that's just dressed up in shiny packaging and empty promises when you can craft your own nutritious and delicious bites with just a handful of wholesome ingredients?

First things first, let's dive into the world of ingredients. You absolutely don't need to be a Michelin-star chef to whip up these delightful bites that everyone will love. Start by grabbing some oats, nut butter, honey, and whatever mix-ins your heart desires that excite you the most. Think about adding chocolate chips, dried fruits, or even a sprinkle of sea salt, as those little additions can transform your creation from "meh" to "wow!" in mere seconds. The best part? You can simply throw everything into a bowl, mix it up as if you're conducting a grand orchestra, and then roll the mixture into bite-sized balls while pretending you're the star of your very own cooking show. Who knew that meal prep could be so entertaining and fun? Enjoy the process and let your creativity shine!

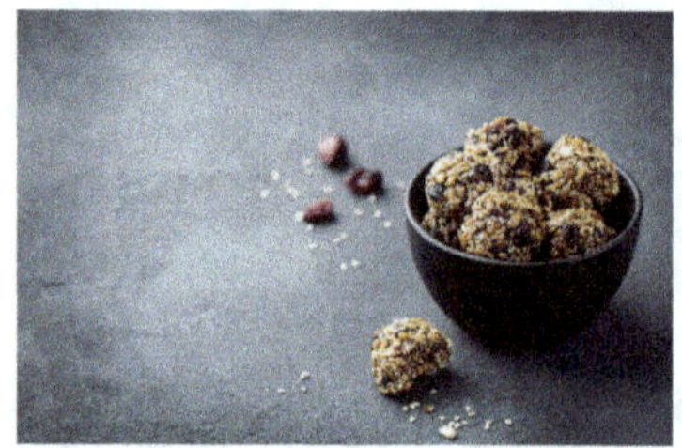

Now, let's address the elephant in the room: the relentless time crunch that so many of us face on a daily basis. Nurses often find themselves running on nothing but caffeine and sheer willpower, which makes the idea of preparing energy bites seem as appealing as enduring a grueling 12-hour shift without so much as a break. But fear not! These energy bites can be whipped up in under 30 minutes, and you'll end up with a generous stash that lasts you all week long. Just imagine it: a no-fuss snack that's ready to go whenever you are, providing you with the energy you need to power through your shifts. Simply toss them in your bag, and you'll have a nutritious pick-me-up at your fingertips that won't require you to sacrifice your last clean scrubs for a bag of chips from the vending machine. Instead, you'll have a delicious, energizing option that fits seamlessly into your hectic schedule, helping you stay fueled and focused, even on the busiest of days.

Storage is another significant advantage for our DIY energy bites. Once you've prepared a batch large enough to feed an army (or at least keep you fueled through those exhausting shifts), you can easily toss them into the fridge or freezer. They'll maintain their shape and flavor much longer than that mysterious meal you accidentally left forgotten in the back of your fridge. Moreover, when the clock strikes 2 AM and your stomach begins to growl louder than a code blue alert, you can simply reach into the fridge and grab a bite without feeling any guilt about your food choices. Enjoy the convenience and peace of mind that comes with having a healthy snack readily available at any hour!

Finally, let's not overlook the immense satisfaction that comes with knowing you've outsmarted the snack industry, which often tries to take advantage of our cravings. Every time you pop one of those delicious energy bites into your mouth, you can't help but chuckle at the thought of how much money you've saved while simultaneously nourishing your body with wholesome ingredients. So, wave goodbye to those overpriced impostors that do little for your health and say a hearty hello to your new favorite snack. With just a bit of creativity, a sprinkle of humor, and a willingness to experiment, you'll soon become a DIY energy bite guru in no time at all, ready to tackle those long night shifts like the superhero you truly are!

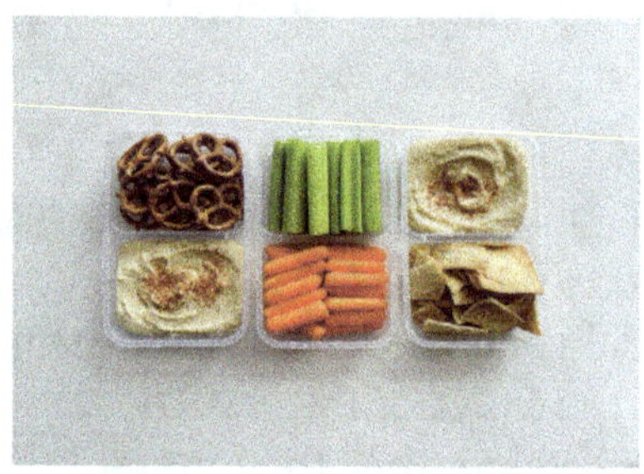

Hydration Station: Staying Refreshed Without the Fancy Labels

When it comes to staying properly hydrated, let's be honest: the fancy labels on bottled water can often make us feel like we need an advanced degree in marketing just to select a simple drink. But here's a little secret—water is fundamentally water, whether it flows from a pristine mountain spring or comes straight from your kitchen tap. As busy nurses, we certainly don't have the time or energy to decipher the nuanced differences between terms like "artisanal" and "filtered." Instead, let's embrace the delightful simplicity of hydration and keep it refreshingly straightforward. We don't need a label that sounds like a luxurious high-end perfume to validate our choice; the essence of hydration is much more important than that.

Imagine this: you're stuck on a grueling 12-hour shift, and the only obstacle between you and a much-needed refreshing drink is a fancy bottle that costs more than your entire lunch. You definitely don't need that kind of unnecessary stress in your life. Instead, grab a reusable water bottle, fill it up from the tap, and toss in a few slices of lemon or cucumber for an extra touch of flavor. Voilà! You've instantly transformed your plain H2O into a delightful spa day experience that feels luxurious. Just make sure you don't accidentally reach for the pickle jar for flavoring—there's a very fine line between refreshing and what you'll ultimately regret. Enjoy your hydration without the added hassle!

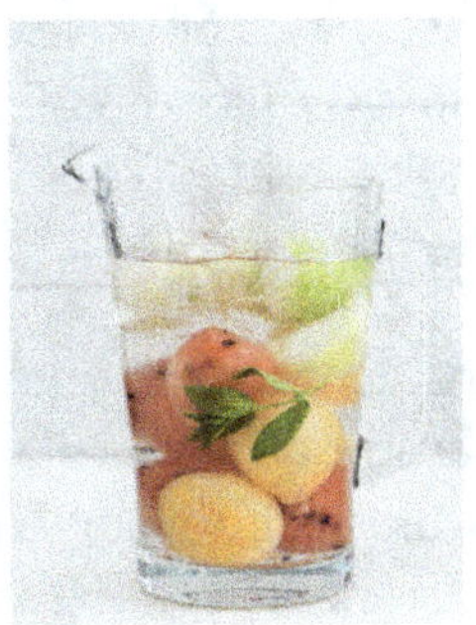

For those long, sleepless night shifts, hydration can often take a backseat to that trusty cup of caffeine. While coffee is truly the lifeblood of countless nurses, it's essential to remember that your body thrives on water as well. Make it a fun game: for every cup of coffee you consume, reward yourself with a refreshing glass of water. It's like a hydration lottery, where the ultimate prize is feeling somewhat human instead of resembling a walking zombie. Not only will this help you maintain your energy levels, but your coworkers will certainly appreciate your newfound vitality—unless, of course, it means you'll be serenading them with show tunes at 3 AM, which could lead to a different kind of midnight madness!

Budget-conscious nursing students, this one's especially for you. Hydration doesn't have to put a strain on your wallet. Instead of shelling out for overpriced flavored waters that can drain your budget faster than you can say "thirsty," get creative with your very own hydration station at home. Start by stocking up on frozen fruits like berries, pineapple, or mangoes; simply toss them into your water, and watch as they transform your drink into a colorful concoction that screams "I'm fancy and refreshing!" all while costing significantly less than a single cup of coffee from a trendy café. Your wallet will truly thank you for this savvy choice, and you'll effortlessly rise to the status of the hydration guru in the break room.

Lastly, let's dive into the engaging topic of snacks. Staying hydrated is not solely about drinking ample amounts of water; it also involves consuming a variety of foods that contribute to a refreshing feeling of energy and vitality. Consider incorporating an array of crunchy veggies that you can dip into creamy hummus or smooth, delicious yogurt. These snacks not only help hydrate your body but also provide the essential fuel needed to tackle whatever chaos your shift throws your way, whether it's a sudden rush of patients or a long stretch of unending tasks.

So, let's set aside those pretentious labels and instead opt for a crisp, satisfying carrot stick or even some colorful bell peppers. Let's hydrate like the dedicated nurses we are—because who truly needs fancy bottled water when you can enjoy a snack that's as invigorating and satisfying as a well-deserved day off? Embrace the simplicity and nourishment of healthy snacks that keep us energized throughout our busy days

Meal Prep Strategies for the Overwhelmed Nurse

05

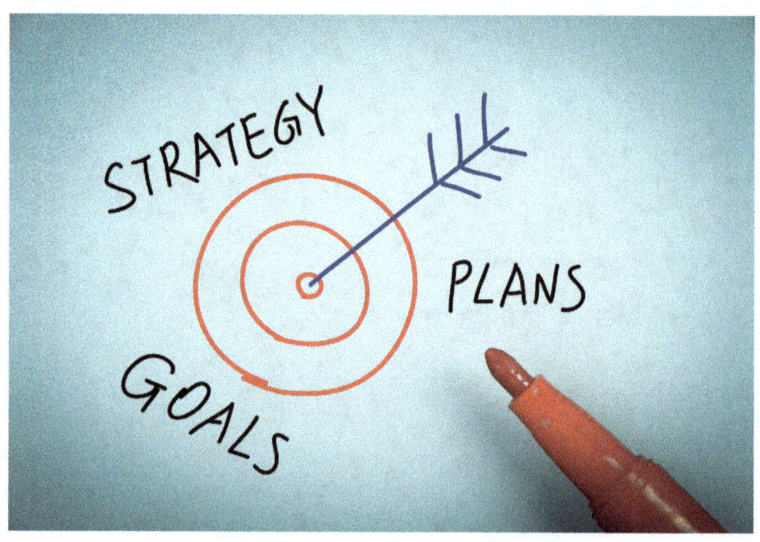

The Sunday Session: How to Make the Most of Your Day Off

The Sunday session is like that precious golden hour before the Monday madness begins, a rare oasis of calm in the whirlwind of life. For busy nurses, it's a sacred time when you can truly recharge your batteries, fill up your fridge with nutritious and delicious grub, and perhaps even enjoy an uninterrupted moment in the bathroom—because let's face it, that's an absolute luxury in your demanding world. Embrace this day off as a golden opportunity to be the culinary superhero you were always meant to be! Don your favorite apron, toss on that 'I'm not on call' t-shirt, and prepare to transform your kitchen into a meal prep haven that would impress even Gordon Ramsay, raising an eyebrow in approval and admiration (in a good way, of course). This is your time to shine, so make it count!

First things first, let's dive into your shopping list. This truly is not the ideal time to test your memory skills—unless you want to find yourself with three jars of pickles and an empty fridge devoid of actual food. Channel your inner nurse and create a meticulously organized list that would earn you an A+ in the art of planning. Focus on quick and easy recipes that can be prepared faster than you can say "stat!" Consider making big batches of chili, hearty and satisfying soups, or a zesty quinoa salad that can happily survive the entire week in your fridge. Remember, low-budget meals don't have to mean bland or boring. With just a little creativity and a sprinkle of imagination, you can transform those canned beans into a vibrant fiesta that even your taste buds will celebrate with joy.

Once you get home, it's time to engage in some serious meal prep that will set you up for a successful week ahead. And by "meal prep," I don't mean just hastily throwing a bunch of takeout containers in the fridge and calling it a day, which is anything but effective. Instead, get those ingredients chopped, roasted, and blended with purpose and enthusiasm! If you're feeling particularly ambitious and want to elevate your organization game, try labeling your containers with the days of the week. Nothing screams "I have my life together" quite like a fridge bursting with neatly labeled meals, each one ready to grab and go. Just don't be surprised when your colleagues start approaching you, eager to ask for your meal prep secrets. It's almost as if you've transformed into the Pinterest guru of the nursing world overnight, inspiring others with your newfound culinary prowess!

And let's not forget about those high-energy snacks that are essential for those marathon shifts. You know the ones—when you're running on caffeine and sheer willpower, trying to make it through the day. It's a great idea to make a big batch of energy balls or some delicious homemade granola bars to keep your energy levels up. You can even get creative with flavors: think chocolate peanut butter, coconut almond, or even "whatever was in the pantry" that you can mix and match. Just make sure to pack them in your bag like the resourceful nurse version of a squirrel preparing for winter, storing up for those long hours ahead. Trust me, your co-workers will be asking you where you bought them, and you can smile knowingly, saying, "Oh, these? Just a little Sunday magic I whipped up in the kitchen."

Finally, take a moment to truly enjoy your day off. This is your well-deserved time to indulge in some much-needed self-care—whether it's binge-watching that show everyone's been raving about or finally diving into that book that's been gathering dust on your nightstand for far too long. And don't forget to treat yourself by putting your feet up with a healthy snack in hand. After all, a well-fed nurse is undoubtedly a happy nurse! So go ahead, savor those precious moments, and keep in mind that while meal prep is undeniably important, your sanity and joy are ultimately the ultimate goals to strive for. Now, go forth and conquer those shifts ahead of you with a full belly and a heart brimming with laughter! Enjoy every bit of your well-earned relaxation!

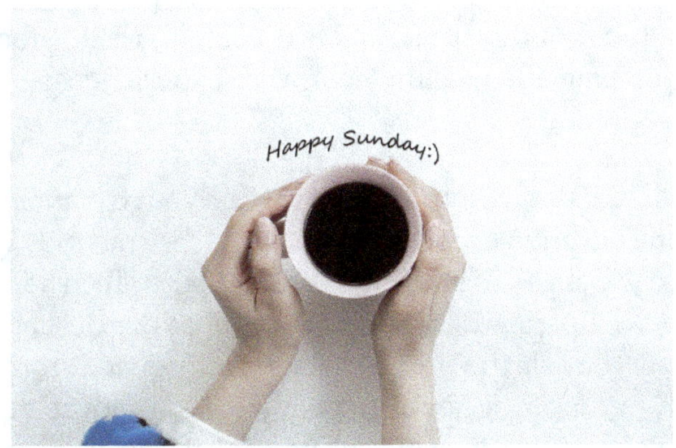

Batch Cooking: Cooking Once, Eating Twice (or Thrice!)

Batch cooking might just be the superhero of meal prep, swooping in to save the day for busy nurses who are constantly juggling their demanding schedules. Picture this: you finally arrive home after an exhausting 12-hour shift, your feet aching and protesting louder than a patient in distress, and the last thing on your mind is the thought of starting to cook a meal from scratch. But fear not! With the magic of batch cooking, you can effortlessly prepare a large quantity of delicious food in one go, allowing you to enjoy not just one meal, but two or even three without having to lift a finger each time. It's like a preemptive strike against hunger, offering you a convenient solution that saves you time and energy. Let's be honest, no one wants to face the daunting prospect of a ravenous stomach after a long, grueling shift. Having that ready-to-eat food waiting for you is a game changer, transforming the post-work experience from stressful to satisfying.

First things first, let's dive into strategy. When you're planning your batch cooking adventure, consider meals that are not only versatile but also have the ability to stand the test of time, both in flavor and in your fridge. Soups, stews, and casseroles are your best allies in this endeavor. They can be prepared in a large pot and stored conveniently in your fridge or even your freezer, ready to be reheated whenever you find yourself in need of a delicious and nutritious meal. Just picture coming home after a long day to a hearty lentil stew that's been patiently waiting for you like a loyal puppy, eager to provide comfort and satisfaction. It truly is a win-win situation: you save precious time during your busy week, and your taste buds get to enjoy a delightful culinary experience.

Now, let's dive into some quick and easy recipes that even a sleep-deprived nurse can whip up with minimal effort! Imagine preparing a giant batch of quinoa salad – it's truly like having a buffet right in a bowl. Simply toss in a variety of colorful veggies, some nutritious beans, and a dressing that makes your taste buds dance with joy. You can enjoy it cold straight from the fridge or heat it up if you prefer a warm meal. And let's not overlook the beauty of stir-fries! They are incredibly fast to make, bursting with color, and can be easily customized with whatever leftover ingredients you have in your fridge. Just keep in mind, the only thing that should be on fire in your kitchen here is your enthusiasm for cooking, not the food itself!

For those nights when you find yourself in need of a tasty snack that truly packs a punch, batch cooking some high-energy snacks can be an absolute game changer. Energy balls made from wholesome oats, creamy nut butter, and a dash of rich chocolate can be prepared in just a matter of minutes, and they'll keep you fueled and energized during those long marathon shifts. Simply roll them up into bite-sized balls, pop them in the fridge, and you'll have a delicious treat that's ready to go whenever you need it. It's like having your very own secret stash of energy—ideal for those moments when you crave an extra boost to help you power through the final hour of your shift. With these handy snacks on hand, you'll be able to maintain your energy levels and stay focused, making even the toughest nights feel a bit more manageable.

Finally, let's not forget about the budget, which is a crucial consideration for any nursing student. Batch cooking is like a financial hug for those navigating the challenges of school while trying to avoid dire financial choices, like selling a kidney. By preparing large quantities of meals in advance, you not only save money but also significantly reduce food waste, all while ensuring that you can enjoy healthy, nutritious food. Plus, who doesn't love the incredible satisfaction that comes from knowing you're feasting on your own homemade creations? So grab those pots and pans, unleash your inner chef, and let batch cooking transform your kitchen into a delightful haven of deliciousness. Your future self will be immensely grateful for the effort, and your taste buds will undoubtedly be throwing an unforgettable party in celebration!

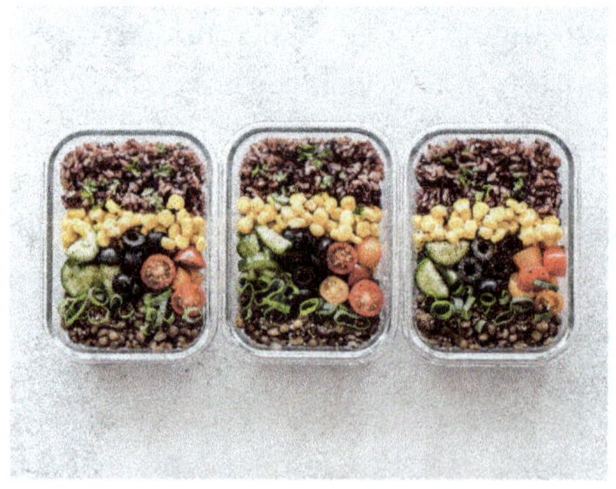

Partner in Crime: Get Your Coworkers to Join the Meal Prep Party

When it comes to meal prep, why go through the process alone when you can easily recruit your coworkers to join in on the fun? After all, misery loves company, and let's be honest, meal prepping can sometimes feel like a punishment even worse than enduring a night shift without a single drop of coffee. Just imagine this scenario: a lively group of dedicated nurses huddled around a spacious table, chopping fresh veggies, sharing hearty laughs, and engaging in a spirited debate about the merits of kale versus spinach. It's like a cooking show, but with a lot more caffeine, plenty of camaraderie, and far fewer commercials to interrupt the action. So grab those scrubs, roll up your sleeves, and let's transform this kitchen into a vibrant culinary battleground where creativity and teamwork collide!

First things first, you need to convince your fellow nurses that meal prep is truly the best thing since sliced bread—preferably whole grain for that added fiber and health boost. Start by presenting the enticing promise of saving time during those chaotic shifts. Who wouldn't want to swap out a frantic dash to the vending machine for a delicious, nourishing homemade quinoa salad packed with fresh veggies? Imagine the joy and relief on their faces when they realize they can actually enjoy something that doesn't resemble a science experiment gone wrong from the depths of the break room fridge. To spice things up, a little friendly competition never hurt anyone, so why not propose a fun "Meal Prep Showdown"? The winner takes home the coveted bragging rights (and maybe some tasty leftovers), making meal prep not just a healthy choice but also an engaging and social experience.

Next, make it a social event. Why not transform those meal prep sessions into a lively potluck? Each nurse can bring along their favorite dish, and just like that, you have a delightful buffet of healthy options that could make even the pickiest eater swoon with joy. It's important to remind everyone that "healthy" doesn't equate to bland or tasteless. A little spice can elevate a dish significantly—unless, of course, you're dealing with someone who believes that black pepper is the height of culinary adventure. Just be ready for the inevitable and friendly debate over whether hummus is classified as a snack or a full meal. Spoiler alert: it can definitely be both if you indulge in enough of it!

Let's not forget the critical budget-friendly angle that resonates deeply with nursing students. Often living on a diet of ramen and coffee, it's essential to show them how effective meal prepping can significantly save their wallets while also providing nutritious options. Consider creating a group chat dedicated specifically to sharing budget-friendly recipes that don't require them to take out a second mortgage on their homes. In addition to main meals, throw in a few high-energy snacks that can be easily consumed during those grueling shifts—think DIY trail mix or energy balls that are delicious yet won't send you spiraling into a sugar coma. By transforming your team into savvy, budget-conscious meal preppers, you will not only save money, but you will also foster a sense of camaraderie and connection as you bond over the common struggles of living paycheck to paycheck, all while cultivating healthier eating habits that can support their demanding lifestyle.

Finally, celebrate your collective and collaborative efforts with an exciting "Meal Prep Party." This event is not merely an excuse to enjoy some delicious food, but it also serves as a fantastic opportunity to share valuable tips, clever tricks, and perhaps even some entertaining kitchen disasters that may have occurred along the way. Make it abundantly clear that this gathering is a judgment-free zone—burnt quinoa, lumpy smoothies, and overambitious Pinterest fails are all more than welcome here. Take the time to share the triumphs of the week, like that moment when you finally mastered the delicate art of cooking brown rice to perfection. At the end of the day, meal prepping with your coworkers transcends just saving time or cutting calories; it's fundamentally about fostering a supportive community that helps you feel less like a solitary wolf and more like a vital part of a well-fed and thriving pack. So now, go forth and transform your meal prep into a lively celebration, because if anyone truly deserves a good time, it's the dedicated nurses who keep the world running smoothly!

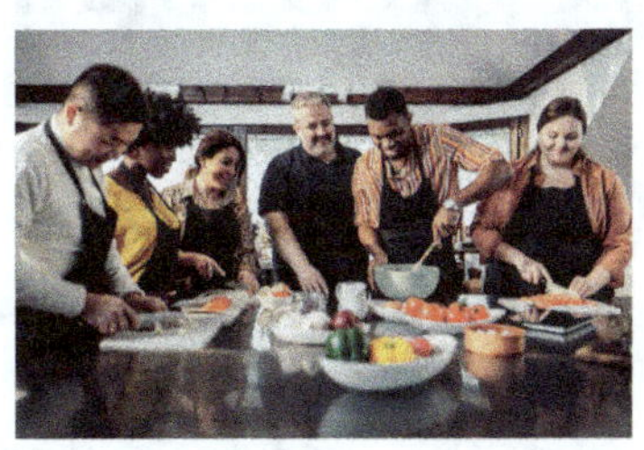

06

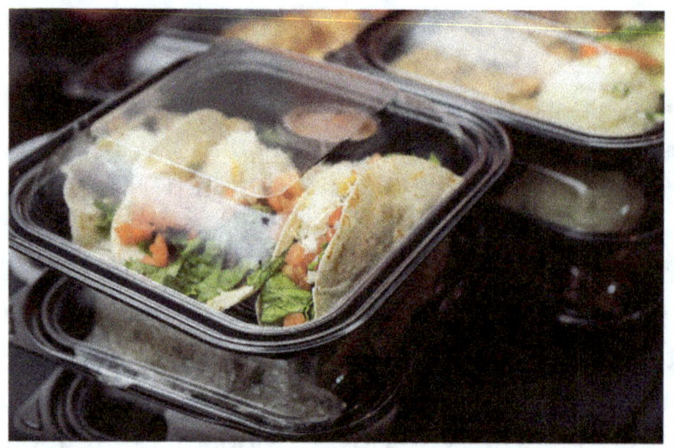

The Art of Eating
Well on the Go

Portable Meals: Tupperware's Time to Shine

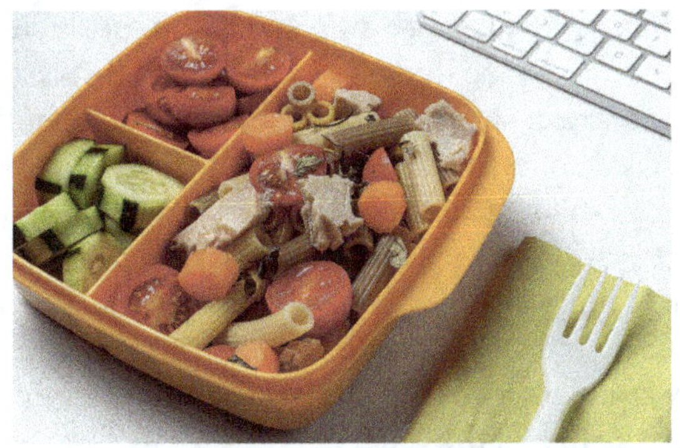

Portable meals are the unsung heroes of the nursing world, transforming every chaotic shift into an exciting culinary adventure filled with flavors and satisfaction. Imagine a world where your lunch doesn't resemble a science experiment that was forgotten in the depths of the fridge for far too long, growing increasingly unrecognizable as the days go by. Enter Tupperware, those magical containers that not only promise to keep your food fresh and delicious but also play a crucial role in preserving your sanity, all while saving you from the curious side-eyes of your colleagues directed at your suspicious leftovers that have seen better days. With the right selection of portable meals, you can confidently conquer both your hunger and the hospital cafeteria's baffling mystery meat, ensuring you stay nourished, satisfied, and energized throughout your demanding shifts, ready to tackle whatever challenges come your way.

First up, let's dive into a conversation about the absolutely glorious creation known as the "nurse's salad." Now, before you roll your eyes and conjure up images of limp lettuce and sad, lifeless tomatoes, let's really spice things up and elevate this dish. We're talking about a vibrant salad that could easily win a beauty pageant —imagine an array of colorful veggies, protein-packed beans, and a dressing that doesn't taste like pure regret. Layer them thoughtfully in your Tupperware with the flair of a culinary Picasso, and you'll have something that not only fuels your energy throughout the day but also makes your coworkers green with envy. Who knew that being healthy could also turn you into the star of the break room and make you the talk of the office?

But wait, there's even more to consider! If salads aren't exactly your jam, how about trying the ultimate pasta salad instead? This definitely isn't your grandma's bland elbow macaroni that you might remember. We're talking about a vibrant and colorful mix of whole grain pasta, perfectly roasted veggies, and just the right dash of Italian dressing that'll have you twirling your fork like a seasoned pro. Best of all, it holds up beautifully in Tupperware, making it incredibly easy for you to take it along on those all-too-frequent night shifts at work. Just make sure to label it clearly—"Not for sharing" might be a wise choice, especially when you catch your colleagues eying it like it's the last delicious donut in the break room, creating a sense of urgency that you'll want to avoid!

Now, let's not forget about the incredible power of snacks. When the clock strikes 3 a.m. and you find yourself battling the overwhelming urge to take a nap on the supply cart, having high-energy snacks readily available can truly be a game changer. Imagine grabbing some portable energy bites that are not only packed with wholesome nuts and hearty oats but also infused with a delightful hint of chocolate—yes, please! Just pop them into your trusty Tupperware, and you'll instantly transform into the superhero of the night shift, zipping around with a burst of energy while your coworkers struggle to keep their eyes open and stay awake. Who says you can't enjoy your snacks and indulge in them at the same time?

Finally, let's not overlook the fantastic budget-friendly options available for our hardworking nursing students. It's time to show those ramen noodles who's really in charge. With Tupperware, you can easily whip up a generous batch of hearty chili or nutritious vegetable soup that not only warms your soul but also provides relief for your wallet. Portion it out into convenient servings, freeze what you don't consume right away, and voilà! You'll have a well-stocked pantry full of portable meals that are ready to save the day —and your budget. So, embrace the Tupperware revolution wholeheartedly, and get ready to nourish yourself and flourish through every demanding shift, one delicious portable meal at a time. Your future self will thank you for these thoughtful preparations.

Snack Packs: The Ultimate Survival Kit for Your Scrubs

Snack packs are the unsung heroes of the nursing realm, standing by like loyal sidekicks when hunger strikes during a chaotic shift. Let's face it, there's nothing worse than the sinking realization that the vending machine has become your only source of sustenance, offering stale chips and candy bars that have certainly seen better days. A well-prepared snack pack can truly save you from the clutches of mid-shift starvation, providing the essential fuel you need to keep your energy levels high and your spirits even higher. These convenient little bundles of nourishment can include a variety of healthy options, ensuring that you have something delicious to reach for when you need it most. Whether it's a handful of nuts, some fresh fruit, or yogurt, a thoughtful assortment can make all the difference in maintaining your focus and stamina throughout those demanding hours on the floor.

Imagine this: it's 3 a.m., you're knee-deep in charting, and your stomach starts growling louder than a code blue alarm ringing through the halls. You could reach for that last slice of pizza you swore you'd save for later, a tempting reminder of the deliciousness you indulged in earlier, or you could unzip your trusty snack pack and unveil a treasure trove of nutritious goodies just waiting to be devoured. Think of it as a portable buffet of delightful bites – from homemade granola bars that won't break the bank and provide the perfect energy boost to veggie sticks paired with a creamy hummus that will make you feel like a health guru instead of a frazzled nurse drowning in paperwork. Who would have thought that carrot sticks could turn into your best friends during a long night shift, providing not just crunch, but also a sense of vitality and refreshment when you need it most?

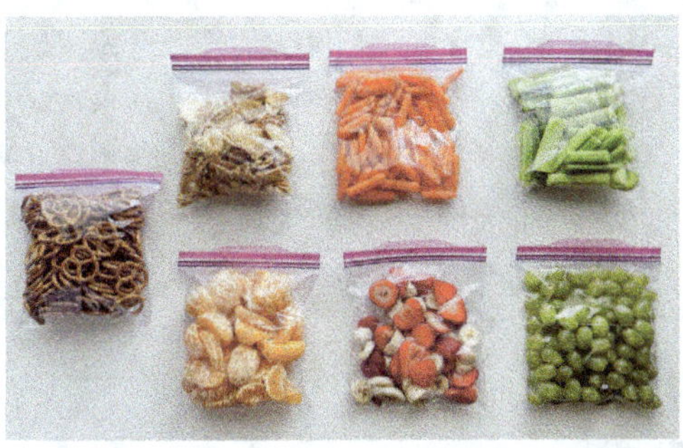

Now, let's dive into the importance of variety because no one wants to be the nurse who's known for munching on the same sad trail mix every single night. It's time to mix it up! One night, you could pack some crisp apple slices paired with smooth almond butter; the next, switch things around and try creamy yogurt cups topped with a delightful sprinkle of granola. For an extra protein boost, you can even throw in some protein-packed boiled eggs, but be cautious of the smell that might waft through the break room – you might need to clear out the space faster than you can utter the words "nurse's lunch break." By infusing a little humor into your culinary creativity, you'll transform your snack packs into not just functional meals but also a source of joy and fun!

Preparing these snack packs doesn't need to be an Olympic event that requires extensive planning and time. We're talking about a quick, easy assembly process that even a sleep-deprived nursing student can manage effortlessly between busy classes and demanding clinicals. Set aside just a few minutes each week to whip up these delicious snacks, and soon you'll find yourself becoming the envy of the break room. Your colleagues will marvel at your impressive organizational skills while they're stuck munching on stale, day-old donuts, and you can graciously hand out your delightful, homemade creations. Just be prepared for the inevitable requests for your "secret recipes," as everyone will want to know your secret to snack success!

In the end, snack packs truly become your very best friends in the demanding world of nursing. They provide you with the essential nourishment needed to successfully tackle your long and often exhausting shifts without having to resort to less-than-ideal options that might leave you feeling sluggish. With a bit of thoughtful planning and a sprinkle of creativity, you can easily transform those hectic and busy hours into a delightful culinary adventure that not only keeps you well-fed but also fuels your enduring passion for patient care. So, wholeheartedly embrace the snack pack movement; your stomach will undoubtedly thank you for it, and your fellow nurses might just start seeing you as their new go-to food guru, eager to share your innovative snack ideas and tips!

Quick Fixes: Emergency Meals for When You're Running Late

When the clock is ticking down and your scrubs are still crumpled and wrinkled from that exhausting 12-hour shift, the very last thing you want to think about is what to make for dinner. Fear not, dear nurse, for the wonderful world of emergency meals is here to rescue you from your culinary despair. Picture this: you walk into your kitchen after a long day, and it resembles a scene from a disaster movie, with dishes piled high and ingredients scattered everywhere. Not to worry! With just a few essential pantry staples and a dash of creativity, you can whip up something delicious that will not only fill your belly but also keep you alert and energized through that demanding night shift. Cue the dramatic music; it's time for "Quick Fixes: Emergency Meals for When You're Running Late." Get ready to transform your kitchen chaos into a satisfying meal in no time!

First up, let's dive into the world of the beloved canned beans. These little legumes are nothing short of the superheroes of your pantry, ready to save the day when you need a quick meal. Toss them into a pot along with some diced tomatoes, chopped onions, and whatever spices you can find that haven't expired yet—this is your chance to get creative! Let it all simmer together while you take a moment to catch your breath, and voilà! You've got a quick chili that's as hearty and satisfying as your determination to survive yet another demanding shift. Serve it over a generous helping of rice or alongside some crunchy tortilla chips, and suddenly, you're not just a nurse; you've transformed into a gourmet chef in disguise. Bonus points if you manage to spill some on your scrubs—just wear those stains like a badge of honor, a testament to your culinary prowess in the midst of a busy day!

If you find yourself racing against the clock and those frozen veggies are staring at you as if they've seen better days, it's definitely time to take decisive action! Grab a frying pan, pour in a generous splash of oil, and toss in those frozen beauties without hesitation. While they're sizzling away and filling your kitchen with delightful aromas, take a moment to grab some eggs and whisk them with enthusiasm like your life truly depends on it (because, let's be honest, it kind of does). Once you've achieved that perfect frothy consistency, pour those eggs over the veggies in the pan and watch the culinary magic unfold before your eyes. In less time than it takes to rummage through your bag to find your favorite pen, you'll have a vibrant and colorful veggie scramble that boldly screams, "I'm healthy and I totally have my life together!" Just don't forget to sprinkle a generous amount of cheese on top—because we all know cheese makes everything better and adds that extra delicious touch!

Now, let's not forget the incredible power of the sandwich. Yes, the classic meal that has saved us all from hunger at one point or another in our busy lives. But we're not just talking about any ordinary sandwich; we're elevating this beloved dish to an art form that deserves celebration. Start by slapping together some hearty whole-grain bread, then add some leftover protein from last night's dinner (because really, who has time to cook every single day?), and finish it off with any random condiments that you can find lurking in the depths of your fridge. Don't forget to throw in some fresh greens for a delightful pop of color and a satisfying crunch. You may find yourself channeling your inner sandwich artist, crafting a masterpiece that could rival those on culinary Pinterest boards—if only in your own imagination.

Finally, let's not overlook the incredible magic of high-energy snacks. As nurses, we know that a well-timed snack can truly make the difference between a productive shift filled with energy and a couch potato moment that leaves us feeling sluggish. So, raid your pantry for an assortment of nuts, seeds, and dried fruit, and toss them into a bowl with the enthusiasm of preparing for a food fight. If you're in the mood for something a bit fancier, add some dark chocolate chips to the mix, and just like that, you've created a delightful trail mix that will keep your energy up and spirits high during those long hours at work. Just remember to store this tasty treat somewhere safe and secure, or you might find yourself unwittingly sharing it with your co-workers—who, let's be honest, will probably devour it faster than you can even say "where did my snacks go?" It's a wild nursing world out there, so keep your snacks close and your energy closer!

So there you have it, some quick and effective fixes for emergency meals that will keep you nourished and energized, even when your schedule feels like an exhilarating rollercoaster ride. With a generous dash of humor and a sprinkle of creativity, you can transform those late-night kitchen panic attacks into delicious culinary triumphs that will satisfy your cravings. Now, go forth and conquer those demanding shifts, armed with your newfound culinary prowess and confidence—because if you can successfully handle the chaos of nursing, you can absolutely tackle a few quick meals with ease and flair!

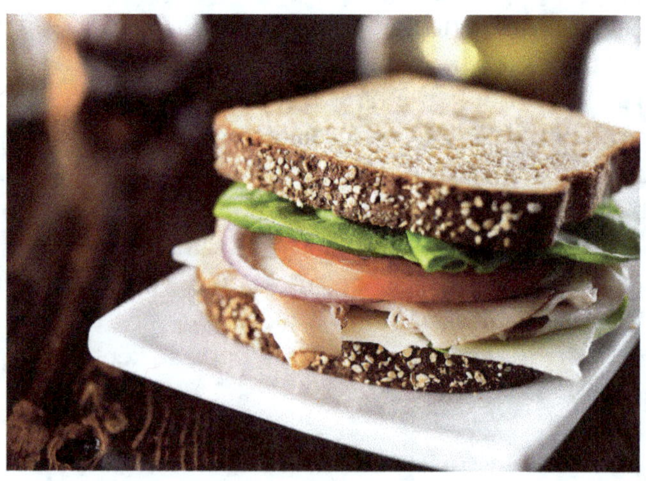

Spice It Up: Flavorful Additions to Keep You Interested

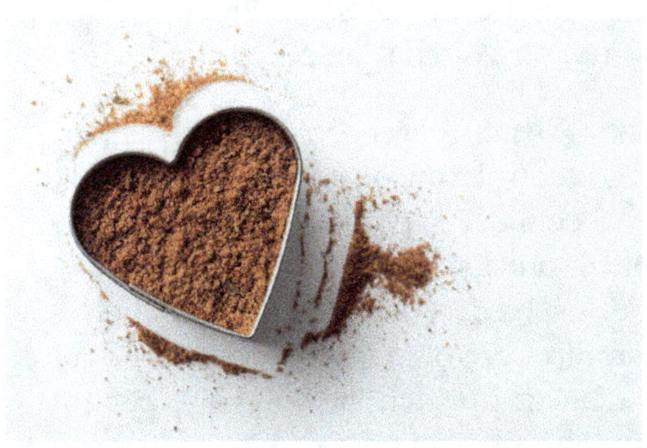

07

Seasoning Secrets: Transform Your Meal from Meh to Marvelous

Seasoning is like the magic wand of the culinary world, turning a bland meal into something that could make your taste buds dance like they just won the lottery. For busy nurses, who often find themselves juggling night shifts and meal preps like a circus performer, knowing how to season your food can be the difference between a "meh" dinner and a "marvelous" one. Imagine coming home after a grueling 12-hour shift, only to be greeted by the aroma of chicken that tastes like it spent the day in the waiting room. No, thank you! Let's sprinkle some spice on that situation.

First up, let's talk about the holy trinity of seasonings: salt, pepper, and garlic. These three amigos can elevate any dish from "what did I just eat?" to "wow, can I have seconds?" A pinch of salt enhances flavor, pepper adds a little kick, and garlic? Well, garlic is basically the fairy godmother of food. Just be careful not to overdo it unless you're trying to ward off vampires or your co-workers. A good rule of thumb is to start light and build up, much like how you'd pace yourself during a night shift coffee marathon.

Next, don't underestimate the power of herbs! Fresh or dried, they are like the superheroes of the seasoning world. Basil, thyme, and rosemary are not just for impressing your friends at a dinner party; they can transform a simple vegetable sauté into a gourmet experience. For those busy evenings, try throwing a handful of

Italian seasoning into your pasta or a dash of cumin into your beans. Your taste buds will be sending you thank-you cards, while your wallet remains untouched because dried herbs are budget-friendly and last longer than your last pair of scrubs.

Now, let's not forget about the underappreciated role of acids in seasoning. A splash of lemon juice or a dash of balsamic vinegar can cut through the richness of heavy dishes and wake up your palate. It's like giving your meal a refreshing slap in the face—minus the actual slap, of course. This little trick works wonders, especially for those night shifts when your energy levels are lower than the hospital vending machine's selection. One squeeze of citrus can make your chicken feel like it just took a vacation to a tropical island instead of sitting in a cafeteria.

Finally, get adventurous! Don't be afraid to explore seasoning blends from different cultures. A little curry powder can turn your usual stir-fry into a flavorful escapade, and taco seasoning can spice up just about anything—yes, even that leftover quinoa from last week. Experimentation is key because, like nursing, cooking is all about finding what works best for you. So go ahead, channel your inner chef, and get those meals from "meh" to "marvelous." After all, just because you're a busy nurse doesn't mean your meals have to be boring!

Saucy Solutions: Dressings and Dips That Make Everything Better

When it comes to dressing up your meals, let's face it: a bland bowl of greens is about as appealing as a 3 AM shift change. Enter the world of dressings and dips, where a little sauce can turn that sad salad into a vibrant feast. Picture this: you've just finished a long shift, and the most exciting thing in your fridge is a container of leftover kale. Sprinkle on a zesty lemon tahini dressing, and suddenly you're dining in a trendy café instead of a half-hearted attempt at nutrition. It's all about the magic of flavor, and luckily, creating these culinary wonders doesn't require a Michelin star or a culinary degree—just a sense of humor and a few staple ingredients.

When it comes to dressing up your meals, let's face it: a bland bowl of greens is about as appealing as a 3 AM shift change. Enter the world of dressings and dips, where a little sauce can turn that sad salad into a vibrant feast. Picture this: you've just finished a long shift, and the most exciting thing in your fridge is a container of leftover kale. Sprinkle on a zesty lemon tahini dressing, and suddenly you're dining in a trendy café instead of a half-hearted attempt at nutrition. It's all about the magic of flavor, and luckily, creating these culinary wonders doesn't require a Michelin star or a culinary degree—just a sense of humor and a few staple ingredients.

Let's talk ranch. Yes, the creamy classic that has somehow wormed its way into every gathering since the dawn of time. But before you reach for that store-bought bottle, why not whip up a homemade version that won't make your arteries cry? Combine Greek yogurt, a splash of buttermilk, and a handful of herbs, and you've got yourself a dip that not only tastes better but is healthier too! Plus, it's a fantastic way to get some protein while you're munching on those carrot sticks during your break. Just remember to keep it hidden from the salad stealers in the break room—they'll be begging for your secret recipe before you can say "crunchy carrots."

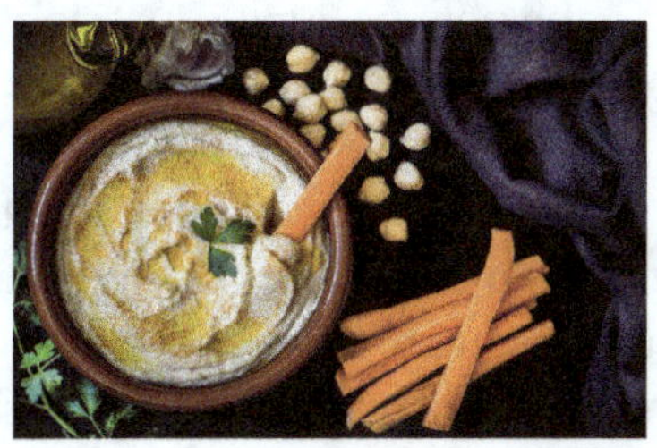

Guacamole is another game changer. You can throw it on tacos, smear it on toast, or just eat it straight with a spoon (no judgment here). To keep it quick and simple, mash up an avocado, squeeze in some lime, and toss in a pinch of salt. Voilà! You've got a dip that brings a fiesta to your meal prep without the need for a mariachi band. And if your night shifts are feeling particularly long, guacamole might just be the emotional support food you didn't know you needed. Just remember, if it starts to turn brown, it's okay —just add a bit more lime juice and pretend it's "rustic."

Now, let's not forget about the power of hummus. This chickpea delight can turn your boring whole-grain crackers into a snack that you'd actually look forward to. Plus, it's a great excuse to load up on those veggies you promised yourself you'd eat more of. Experiment with flavors—roasted red pepper, garlic, or even a spicy harissa version. It's like a flavor party in your mouth, and the best part is, it's super cheap to make. Just throw everything in a blender and let it work its magic. You'll be so proud of this dip that you might even consider bringing it to the next potluck—just don't let the other nurses know how easy it was to make.

Lastly, let's sprinkle some sass into your meals with a homemade vinaigrette. A basic formula of oil, vinegar, and mustard can be your best friend when you're trying to jazz up a boring dish. Experiment with different oils and vinegars to keep things fresh and exciting. A little apple cider vinegar can turn a mundane grain bowl into a tangy delight that will make you forget you're eating a healthy meal. And if you're feeling especially daring, throw in some honey or maple syrup for a sweet twist. Remember, the goal is to make your meals as fabulous as you are, especially after a grueling shift. So go ahead, dress it up, dip it down, and savor every flavorful bite!

Herbs and Spices: The Real MVPs of Your Meal Prep

Herbs and spices are the secret agents of the culinary world, stealthily transforming bland, sad meals into vibrant dishes that even your taste buds will applaud. You know those nights when you're staring at a sad piece of chicken and wondering if you should just give in and order takeout? Enter your trusty herb and spice collection. A sprinkle of garlic powder here, a dash of paprika there, and suddenly you're not just a nurse; you're the Gordon Ramsay of your kitchen. Well, minus the yelling and the British accent, but you get the idea.

Imagine this: it's 3 AM, you're halfway through a twelve-hour shift, and your stomach is growling louder than a code blue. You pull out your prepped meal, and what do you find? A beautifully seasoned quinoa bowl that practically sings "Eat me!" instead of the usual "I'm a sad desk lunch." With a few herbs and spices, you can elevate even the most basic ingredients to gourmet status. Think of basil, your basil. It's like a mini vacation to Italy every time you sprinkle it on your pasta. And we all know that nursing shifts can make you feel like you've been to war, so why not treat your taste buds to a little getaway?

Let's talk budget, because we all know nursing school and working nights don't exactly pay for lavish meals. The beauty of herbs and spices is that they're the culinary equivalent of a magic wand. A small investment in a few basic herbs and spices can turn your low-budget meals into a flavor fiesta. A jar of cumin and some chili flakes can turn your plain rice into a flavorful pilaf that'll have your colleagues asking if you've been moonlighting as a chef. Plus, these flavor boosters last a long time, so it's like having a secret stash of happiness right in your pantry.

And what about those high-energy snacks we all need during those exhausting shifts? Instead of reaching for that vending machine candy, how about some roasted chickpeas sprinkled with a bit of paprika and garlic? Not only will you fuel your body with something wholesome, but you'll also impress everyone with your culinary prowess. You'll be the nurse who transforms ordinary snacks into gourmet delights. Your colleagues will start expecting you to host cooking classes in the break room, and you'll have them all munching on herbed popcorn instead of potato chips in no time.

In a world filled with stress and long hours, herbs and spices are your culinary allies, ready to come to the rescue. They are the MVPs of your meal prep, making your food not only delicious but also a joy to eat. So next time you're planning your meals for the week, don't forget to unleash the power of herbs and spices. They're the unsung heroes of healthy meal prep, and they'll help you nourish and flourish, one delicious bite at a time.

08

Support Your Fellow Nurses: Meal Swap Ideas

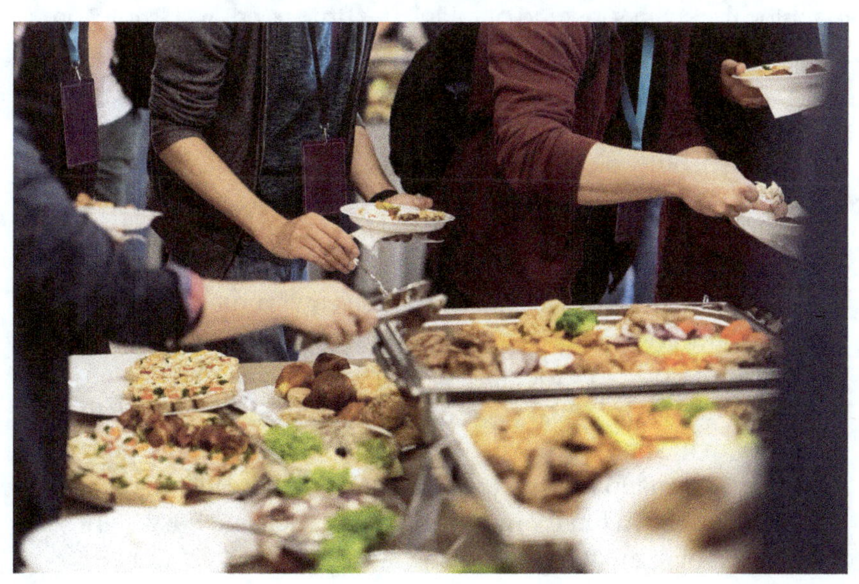

Organizing a Meal Swap: How to Make Friends and Influence Meals

Organizing a meal swap is a lot like hosting a potluck, but with significantly fewer moments of awkward small talk and a greater focus on delicious food. It's truly a win-win situation: you have the opportunity to trade your culinary masterpieces (or perhaps your latest Pinterest fail) for someone else's unique creations, and in the process, you might just forge some new friendships. As busy nurses, we often find ourselves resorting to raiding the hospital vending machine for snacks instead of taking the time to enjoy a wholesome, home-cooked meal. By orchestrating a meal swap, you can fill your fridge with healthy, homemade delights that are both satisfying and nutritious, all while bonding over the shared challenge of trying to maintain a healthy diet amidst our hectic schedules.

First things first, you need to rally your fellow nurses and get everyone excited. Start with some light-hearted banter about the joys of hospital cafeteria food or how you can't remember the last time you had a real meal that didn't come from a vending machine. Use the power of social media, like a fun group chat or a dedicated Facebook event, or even a good old-fashioned bulletin board in the break room to spread the word effectively. Once you have gathered a few willing participants who are on board with the idea, set a date and come up with a fun theme. Maybe it's "Quick and Easy Night Shift Meals" or "Low-Budget Nursing Student Favorites" that everyone can relate to. Whatever theme you choose, just make sure it's something that won't take a PhD in culinary arts to prepare and that everyone can easily contribute to, so no one feels overwhelmed.

Now that you have gathered your crew, it's time to dive into the nitty-gritty details of meal prep! Encourage everyone to unleash their culinary skills and whip up their best dish, but do remind them that we're not trying to impress Gordon Ramsay here. The main goal is to create meals that are not only healthy but also easy to heat up during those chaotic shifts, ensuring that no one ends up searching for a fire extinguisher in the process. Think hearty, comforting soups, delicious casseroles, or even an impressive batch of energy-boosting snacks that can be quickly devoured during a brief break. And don't forget to include a few secret family recipes— everyone truly appreciates a good story behind their food, which can make the meal even more enjoyable and meaningful.

On the day of the swap, be sure to bring your A-game along with a couple of reusable containers to help transport your delicious creations. Set up a vibrant table where everyone can proudly display their culinary masterpieces for all to see. Don't hesitate to sample each other's dishes; this is where the real magic happens! You'll not only have the opportunity to taste a variety of new and exciting recipes but also share invaluable tips and tricks for meal prep that can save you precious time and hard-earned money. Plus, nothing fosters a sense of camaraderie quite like a little friendly competition over who can make the best chili. Spoiler alert: everyone's chili is sure to be the best, especially after a long and exhausting shift! Embrace the fun and creativity of this gathering, and enjoy every moment of it!

As you immerse yourself in the exciting world of meal swapping, remember to keep the atmosphere lighthearted and enjoyable. Share your epic kitchen fails with humor, and don't forget to celebrate all the delicious victories together. Encourage your fellow nurses to enthusiastically exchange recipes and creative meal ideas, fostering a supportive community where everyone lifts each other up, one delightful and nutritious meal at a time. By the end of this event, you'll not only have a fridge brimming with an array of healthy meals but also a newfound appreciation for the culinary skills and creativity of your fellow nurses. Who would have imagined that swapping meals could also lead to the sharing of stories, contagious laughter, and perhaps even the beginning of a few lifelong friendships that enrich your lives both personally and professionally?

Recipes to Share: What to Bring and What to Avoid (No One Needs Your Tuna Casserole)

When it comes to sharing food in the break room or at potluck gatherings, there are definitely some dishes that should make the list while others should be left at home, preferably tucked away under a blanket of shame. Nurses are indeed the unsung heroes of the healthcare system, tirelessly working to care for others, but that doesn't mean we need to endure the unsung horrors of poorly executed tuna casserole or other culinary disasters. Seriously, if your dish emits an aroma that could double as a biohazard in a lab, it's best to take a moment to reconsider what you're planning to bring. Let's face it, we're all exhausted enough after a long shift without having to deal with the puzzling mystery of your so-called "secret ingredient" that might just be better off remaining a mystery forever. After all, the break room should be a place to relax and enjoy good food, not a culinary gamble where we have to question our life choices.

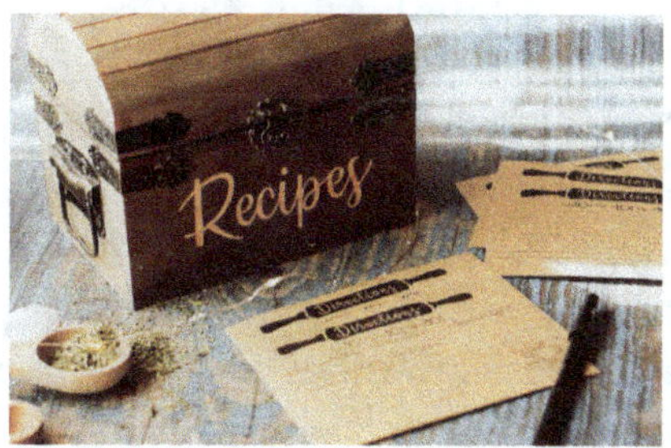

First on the list of what to bring: anything that boldly expresses "I care about your taste buds and the experience of eating." Think fresh salads brimming with vibrant, colorful veggies, or delightful homemade energy bites that might taste like indulgent dessert but are surprisingly packed with wholesome protein. No one wants to open a container only to find a gelatinous mass that bears an unfortunate resemblance to cat food. Instead, why not whip up a delicious quinoa salad with hearty chickpeas and a zesty dressing that dances on the palate? It's not only nutritious and easy to prepare in large quantities, but it also won't make anyone question your culinary sanity or skills. Plus, it serves as a fantastic conversation starter—"Is this a salad or a party in my mouth?" Spoiler alert: it's both, and it's bound to impress everyone at the gathering.

Now, let's dive into the foods you should definitely avoid bringing to your potluck, and tuna casserole is just the tip of the iceberg. If a dish can be served in an emergency room under the guise of diagnosis, it's probably not the best choice for a friendly get-together. Steer clear of overly complicated dishes that require a degree in molecular gastronomy to prepare or even consume. Your coworkers are not prepared for a deconstructed lasagna presented in tiny jars, no matter how trendy that might sound. Keep it simple, keep it tasty, and for the love of all things delicious, please leave the jello salads at home. We all know that no one truly enjoys the peculiar texture of wobbly, neon-colored gelatin, and it's best to avoid any potential culinary disasters that could lead to awkward silence around the table.

For those late-night shifts when energy levels plummet quicker than a dropped stethoscope, it's essential to bring snacks that truly pack a punch. Think about a carefully curated trail mix that skips the mystery fruit bits which often make you question your life choices. Instead, opt for a delightful mix of crunchy nuts, rich dark chocolate, and perhaps a few dried cranberries that won't turn into a sticky mess in your purse or backpack. And let's be honest, who doesn't love a good snack that not only satisfies your cravings but also serves as a much-needed pick-me-up? You'll be the hero of the night shift, the one who brought the good stuff that everyone craves —no one wants to be that person who shows up with a bag of stale chips and a sad, lonely dip that nobody wants to touch. Your thoughtful snack choices will surely elevate the shift and keep everyone energized and happy.

In conclusion, when it comes to sharing recipes among your fellow nurses, keep in mind: make it delightful, ensure it's nutritious, and for the love of all that is holy, let's keep it tuna-free. Embrace the joy of cooking by offering easy, healthy options that won't raise eyebrows or trigger any gag reflexes. Your coworkers will genuinely appreciate your thoughtfulness and culinary skills, and you'll undoubtedly earn the esteemed title of "Nurse Chef Extraordinaire." So go forth and spread the joy of delicious food—just make sure it's not the kind that smells like the bottom of a fish tank. Remember, the kitchen should be a place of creativity and happiness, where every meal brings a smile, not a grimace.

Creating a Meal Prep Community: Because You're All in This Together

Let's face it, nurses are basically superheroes in scrubs, tirelessly battling the challenges of healthcare. However, even the most dedicated superheroes need a reliable sidekick now and then. Enter the vibrant meal prep community, your trusty band of culinary comrades who truly understand the struggle of staying healthy while juggling demanding night shifts, early mornings, and those inevitable late-night caffeine fixes. Picture this: a lively group of exhausted, caffeine-fueled nurses swapping recipes and sharing their most epic meal prep fails over a cup of lukewarm coffee that has seen better days. It's like a support group, but instead of shedding tears over our feelings and hardships, we're laughing and crying over our burnt broccoli disasters, sharing tips and tricks to make our meal prep adventures a little less chaotic and a lot more enjoyable.

In this noble quest for healthy eating, a meal prep community is not merely helpful; it's absolutely essential for anyone looking to improve their culinary skills and nutrition. You'll discover that camaraderie flourishes when you share your triumphs and disasters in the kitchen, creating lasting bonds over food. Did your quinoa turn into a sticky, glue-like substance that seemed impossible to salvage? Don't worry; we've all been there at some point! Grab a fellow nurse, and together, you can laugh it off while devising a foolproof plan to ensure that this culinary mishap never happens again. Plus, there's something incredibly therapeutic and uplifting about bonding over shared kitchen catastrophes and learning from each other's mistakes. After all, the only thing worse than a failed recipe is experiencing it in isolation, without anyone to share the experience or the lessons learned.

Imagine the immense joy of swapping quick and easy recipes, particularly those that can be transformed into a night-shift-friendly feast that keeps your energy up. Your meal prep group can evolve into a treasure trove of innovative ideas for meals that can be thrown together in a pinch, making your late-night cooking a breeze. Who really needs a fancy cookbook when you have a friend who wholeheartedly swears by a five-ingredient chili that saved them from a midnight snack meltdown? You'll become each other's culinary lifeline, exchanging clever hacks for turning last night's leftovers into today's gourmet snack. And just think of the pure satisfaction and pride you'll feel when you serve your colleagues a delicious dish they can't believe was prepped in under 30 minutes! The camaraderie and creativity in the kitchen will elevate your meals to a whole new level, making every shift a delightful experience.

Let's not overlook the dedicated nursing students out there who are working hard to stretch every dollar they have. A meal prep community serves as the ideal platform for sharing creative, low-budget meal ideas that won't cause your wallet to weep. Do you have a hidden stash of ingenious instant ramen hacks that can elevate a simple meal? Or perhaps you've perfected a fantastic recipe for a massive pot of hearty vegetable soup that could feed an entire army, or at least your entire study group? By coming together to pool resources and exchange tips, everyone can enjoy satisfying meals without having to rely solely on a monotonous diet of instant noodles and vending machine snacks. Moreover, there's truly nothing quite like the experience of bonding with friends over a budget-friendly feast that not only fills your stomach but also leaves your taste buds dancing with delight.

Finally, high-energy snacks are truly the lifeblood of any nurse's survival kit, and what better way to keep spirits soaring than by sharing creative snack ideas? Whether it's homemade protein bars bursting with flavor or the infamous "nurse energy bites" that taste surprisingly like dessert, the possibilities for delicious creations are indeed endless. You might even consider hosting a lively snack swap where everyone brings their best culinary creations to share. Just imagine the sheer joy of discovering that your colleague's secret energy bite recipe includes chocolate, making it a delightful treat. In a meal prep community, you're not only nourishing your bodies; you're also fueling friendship, laughter, and perhaps a little healthy competition to see who can craft the best snack. So, gather your fellow nurses, roll up your sleeves, and let's whip up some fun and creativity in the kitchen together! With every bite, you'll be building camaraderie and enjoying the process of creating something special.

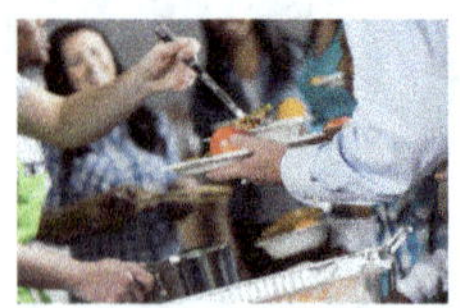

09

Keeping It Real: Nutrition for the Busy Nurse

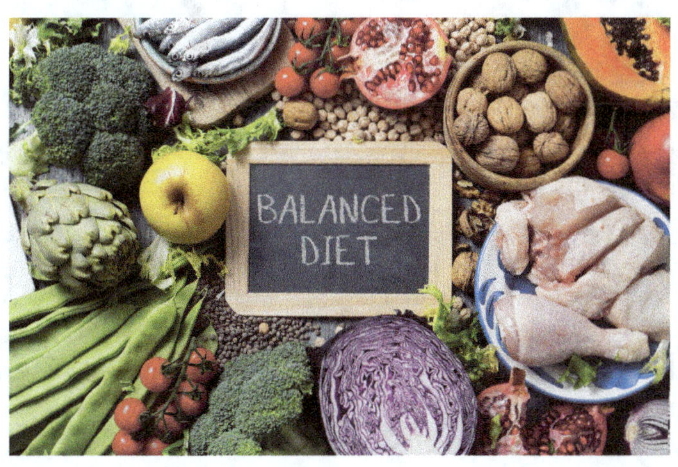

Understanding Your Nutritional Needs: Don't Let Your Stomach Call the Shots

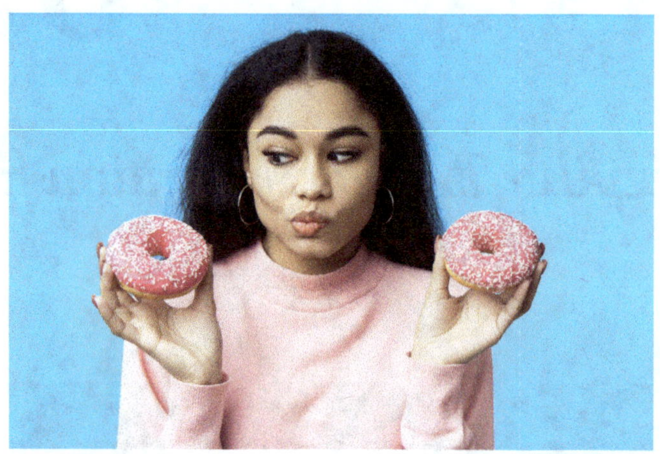

Your stomach has a sneaky way of pulling the strings, especially after a long shift when the only thing you can think about is food. But let's be real; letting your stomach take the wheel is like handing the keys to your car to a toddler. Sure, it might be fun for a minute, but you'll end up somewhere you didn't want to go—with a hefty side of regret. Instead, it's time to take charge of your nutritional needs with a thoughtful plan that doesn't involve succumbing to a vending machine's irresistible siren call or the tempting allure of a midnight pizza delivery. Consider preparing healthy snacks in advance or planning balanced meals that can sustain your energy levels and keep your cravings in check.

First things first, understanding your nutritional needs is akin to knowing your favorite coffee order—absolutely essential for your survival and well-being. As dedicated nurses, you are all too aware of the vital importance of maintaining high energy levels, particularly during those relentless night shifts that can sometimes feel never-ending. Think of your body as a finely tuned engine; it requires the right kind of fuel to operate efficiently and effectively. This means loading up on whole grains, lean proteins, and a vibrant array of colorful fruits and vegetables that nourish your body and keep you energized throughout your demanding shifts. The next time your stomach begins grumbling louder than an alarm clock ringing in a sleepy break room, take a moment to remind yourself that a well-balanced snack is your best ally. It's definitely not the leftover donuts from the last staff meeting that will help you power through!

Now, let's delve into the world of quick and easy meal prep. You might not have the luxury of time to whip up an elaborate gourmet feast after a grueling 12-hour shift, but that certainly doesn't mean your meals can't be both delicious and nutritious at the same time. Batch cooking is truly your secret weapon in this scenario. Take a few hours on your day off to prepare meals that you can effortlessly grab when you're running late or feeling overwhelmed. Consider options like vibrant stir-fries, hearty soups, or refreshing salads that can be thrown together in a matter of minutes. Just like a superhero relies on a trusty cape, you need a solid meal prep strategy to swoop in and save the day when hunger strikes unexpectedly. This approach not only keeps you nourished but also helps you maintain your energy levels and stay focused throughout your busy days.

Budget constraints are a significant reality, especially for nursing students who are working hard to balance their tuition expenses with the rising costs of everyday items like avocados. But fear not! Healthy eating doesn't have to be a financial burden. Instead, embrace the incredible power of legumes, grains, and seasonal produce, which are not only often wallet-friendly but also packed with essential nutrients that your body needs. Plus, buying in bulk can feel like a triumphant victory lap for your wallet, allowing you to save significantly over time. Who knew that being frugal could be so empowering and beneficial for both your health and finances? The next time you're at the store, channel your inner savvy shopper and make it a point to stock up on items that will fill your pantry generously without emptying your pockets. You'll be amazed at how much you can save while still enjoying delicious and nutritious meals!

Finally, let's not forget about snacks. Those high-energy snacks you carefully stash in your scrubs should be as dependable and essential as your trusty stethoscope. It's important to choose options that provide a substantial boost without leaving you feeling heavy or uncomfortable, as if you just swallowed a brick. Consider snacks like a mix of nuts, creamy yogurt, or even homemade energy balls that are packed with nutritious ingredients. These choices will help keep your energy levels stable and your stomach satisfied during those long, grueling shifts that can seem never-ending. So, the next time your stomach tries to lead you astray with cravings for unhealthy options, remember that you have the power to make thoughtful choices. With a bit of planning and a dash of creativity, you can nourish your body effectively and truly flourish in your career—without letting your stomach dictate your snacking decisions!

choices. With a bit of planning and a dash of creativity, you can nourish your body effectively and truly flourish in your career—without letting your stomach dictate your snacking decisions!

Myths and Misconceptions: Debunking the Diet Dilemmas

Myths about diet and nutrition can often become as tangled as the cords on your headphones after a long, demanding shift. One of the most prevalent myths is that healthy eating simply takes too much time. When you envision gourmet meals, it's easy to picture an elaborate three-hour cooking marathon, complete with sophisticated sous-vide gadgets and a stylish chef's hat. However, for busy nurses and healthcare professionals, meal prep can be incredibly straightforward and efficient. It can be as simple as quickly throwing some colorful veggies in a hot pan, adding in a source of protein, and calling it a day. It's important to remember that the only thing that should consume hours of your time is your Netflix binge after a long shift, not the process of preparing your meals. With a little creativity and planning, you can enjoy nutritious food without sacrificing all your free time.

Another popular misconception is that healthy food is always expensive, which many people believe without questioning it. Who decided that quinoa should cost more than a small fortune anyway? The truth is, you can whip up absolutely delicious and nutritious meals on a budget without sacrificing quality or taste. Canned beans, frozen veggies, and seasonal produce are truly your best friends in the kitchen. Think of it as a culinary version of "Survivor," where creativity and resourcefulness will lead you to victory. You'll be amazed at what you can create with just a can of chickpeas and a dream. Plus, your wallet will thank you for making smart choices, and you can save that extra cash for your next coffee run—because let's face it, we all need a little caffeine boost to survive those long and tiring night shifts.

Then there's the common belief that healthy meals are bland and boring. This idea is completely wrong! Eating healthy does not mean you have to sacrifice flavor or enjoyment in your meals. If your dishes taste like cardboard, it's definitely time to spice things up, quite literally. Herbs, spices, and sauces can transform a mundane plate of chicken and broccoli into a vibrant flavor explosion that would earn rave reviews from any food critic. Embrace the art of seasoning and don't be afraid to get creative and experiment with different combinations. Your taste buds will dance with joy at the delightful flavors, and you might just impress your colleagues during lunch break with your newfound culinary prowess. So go ahead, make healthy eating an exciting and delicious adventure!

One of the most laughable myths surrounding meal prepping is the idea that it means you have to consume the same dish every single day. Who honestly wants to eat a week's worth of bland chicken and rice? That sounds more like a punishment than an enjoyable meal plan. The true beauty of meal prep lies in its incredible variety. You can batch-cook a selection of delicious staples and then mix and match them throughout the week to create different combinations. Think of it as a delightful buffet right at your fingertips. One day you might enjoy a flavorful taco bowl, and the next, you could indulge in a vibrant stir-fry. By keeping your meals interesting and diverse, your taste buds will certainly thank you for it, even if your fridge might feel a little overcrowded with all those tempting choices. Embrace the creativity that meal prep offers, and you'll never feel bored with your food again.

Finally, let's tackle the persistent myth that snacking is inherently bad. As nurses, we understand that those long, demanding shifts can often lead to hunger pangs that hit harder and more urgently than a caffeine crash on a particularly exhausting day. So, instead of mindlessly reaching for a pack of stale crackers that offer little in terms of nutrition or satisfaction, why not prepare a variety of high-energy snacks that will keep you fueled, focused, and ready to tackle whatever comes your way? Consider options like homemade energy balls packed with nuts and seeds, crunchy veggie sticks paired with creamy hummus, or a delightful mix of yogurt topped with fresh, vibrant fruit. These snacks are not just beneficial for your body; they're also fantastic for your soul—because really, who doesn't love a little snack time to break up the chaos during a hectic shift? Embrace the snack life wholeheartedly, and you'll find yourself powering through those demanding shifts like the superhero you truly are, ready to make a difference in the lives of your patients.

Balance is Key: Treat Yourself Without Guilt (Because Cake is Life)

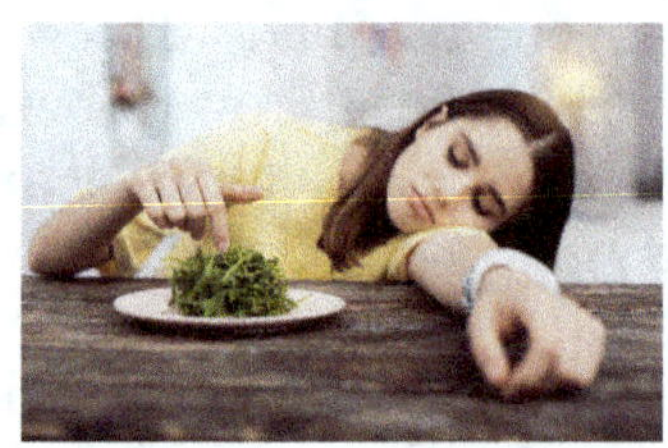

In the chaotic world of nursing, where caffeine is often your best friend and lunch breaks seem like mythological creatures that rarely make an appearance, finding a moment to treat yourself can feel akin to searching for a unicorn in a forest. But here's the undeniable truth: you absolutely deserve that slice of cake, or even two, without a single ounce of guilt weighing you down. After all, if cake is truly life, then let's treat it with the VIP status it rightfully deserves! Embrace the sheer joy of indulging in a delightful sweet treat after a long, exhausting shift, because nothing quite encapsulates the sentiment of "I survived another grueling 12-hour shift" like a forkful of rich chocolate goodness melting in your mouth. So go on, savor that well-earned treat and celebrate your resilience!

Now, let's get real for a moment. You might be thinking, "But I'm supposed to be healthy!" Yes, you absolutely are, but that doesn't mean you can't enjoy a slice of cake while savoring the moment—preferably while wearing scrubs that still fit comfortably. Balance is crucial, especially when you find yourself running on little sleep and even less time for proper self-care. A little indulgence here and there can actually enhance your overall well-being and mental health. Picture this: you've just crushed a demanding night shift, you're utterly exhausted, and the only thing that can truly revive your spirit is a rich, decadent slice of red velvet cake. Embrace that craving! Just think about how happy that little piece of cake must feel to be part of your well-deserved treat, bringing a bit of joy to your busy life.

Let's not forget about those pesky nursing school budgets that can often feel like a heavy weight on our shoulders. You might be living off instant noodles and coffee, but there's always room for a delicious dessert that can brighten your day. Think of it as an essential investment in your mental well-being and sanity. Low-budget meals don't have to mean low-taste or no-fun; in fact, they can be quite the opposite! Create a "treat yourself" fund with spare change from your shifts—it's basically like a self-care savings account that allows you to indulge guilt-free. When the moment arrives for a little indulgence, you can confidently whip out your secret stash of coins and declare, "Cake is a necessity, not a luxury!" Embrace the idea that treating yourself is a crucial part of navigating the challenges of nursing school.

And for those long shifts that feel like they're truly never-ending, high-energy snacks are undoubtedly your best allies. Pair those energizing snacks with a guilt-free dessert to elevate your spirits! A healthy trail mix can keep you fueled throughout the day, but you know what pairs exceptionally well with a handful of almonds? A delightful mini cupcake! It's all about finding that balance in moderation. You can absolutely be the nurse who rocks a healthy lifestyle while also being the one who knows exactly where the best bakery in town is located. In the grand scheme of things, indulging in a little cake isn't going to derail your healthy eating goals; rather, it's just a sweet boost to keep you energized and motivated as you tackle your demanding shifts. Embrace both nutrition and a little indulgence for a well-rounded approach to your day!

So here's the bottom line: life as a nurse is undeniably tough, and you absolutely deserve to celebrate your hard work and dedication. Make it a priority to schedule that cake break with the same fervor and commitment as you would when administering a patient's medication. Finding balance in your life is key, and treating yourself without a hint of guilt is essential to your well-being. So, the next time you find yourself gazing at a delicious slice of cake, remember: you're not just indulging in dessert; you're nourishing your spirit and replenishing your energy. After all, cake is not just a treat; it's a joyful celebration of life, and you, dear nurse, are a true connoisseur of both health and happiness! Enjoy every delightful bite as a reward for all the care you give.

10

The Final Countdown: Meal Prep Success Stories

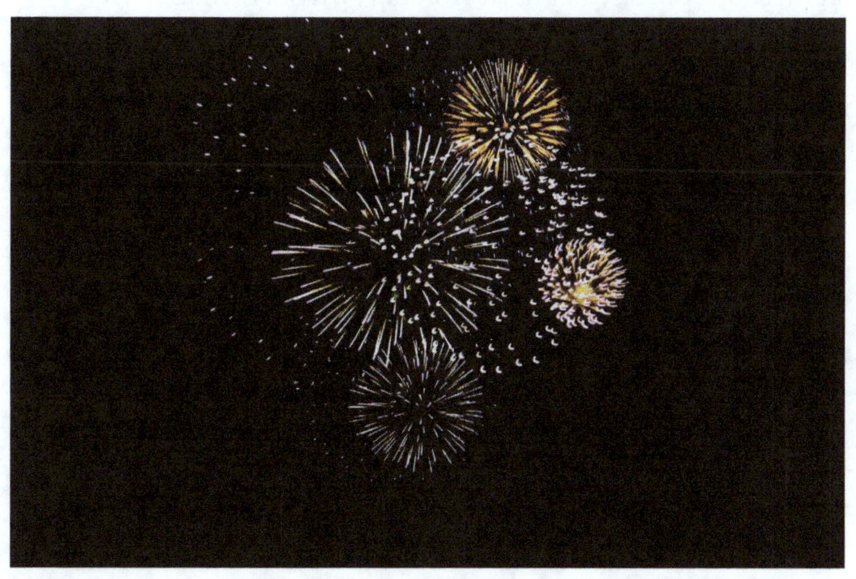

Nurses That Prep: Stories That Will Inspire You

Nursing is a demanding profession, and let's face it, sometimes the only thing keeping us going through those long shifts is the promise of a good meal. Meet Sarah, a night shift warrior who turned her chaotic meal prep into a well-oiled machine. Sarah, armed with her trusty slow cooker and a freezer full of homemade chili, has mastered the art of making meals that can be both delicious and nutritious. One fateful night, after a particularly grueling 13-hour shift, she discovered that her secret weapon was not just her stethoscope but also her ability to whip up a pot of magic. A few batches of chili, and she transformed from a hangry nurse into a chili connoisseur. Now, she tells her friends that her secret ingredient is "survival" and a generous sprinkle of cumin.

Then there's Tom, the nursing student who learned early on that ramen noodles should not be his go-to dinner if he wanted to avoid a life of emergencies in more ways than one. With a tight budget, he got creative with meal prep, utilizing his student discount at the local grocery store like a pro. After a few trial-and-error sessions, Tom discovered the beauty of batch cooking stir-fry. With a week's worth of veggies, rice, and soy sauce, he was able to whip up a colorful plate that not only looked Instagram-worthy but also filled his belly without breaking the bank. Now, he's known as the "Stir-Fry King" among his classmates, and it's safe to say his cooking has saved many a late-night study session.

And let's not forget about Jessica, who made it her mission to create high-energy snacks for those seemingly endless shifts. She realized that granola bars from the vending machine were not cutting it, especially when her energy dipped lower than her patient's blood pressure. With a bit of trial and error (and maybe a few too many attempts at perfecting energy balls), she concocted a recipe for peanut butter oat bites that even the pickiest of coworkers couldn't resist. Now, she walks onto the floor like a snack fairy, armed with Tupperware filled with these little delights, ready to share. Her coworkers have dubbed her "Snackzilla," and her breaks are now the highlight of the night shift.

Then, we have the legendary duo, Mark and Liz, who decided that healthy meal prep could become a competitive sport. They made it their mission to outdo each other with quick and easy recipes. One week, Mark brought in his famous quinoa salad topped with a zesty lemon dressing, while Liz retaliated with a taco bar that would make even Taco Tuesday jealous. Their playful rivalry turned into a meal prep Sunday tradition, inspiring others on their unit to join in the fun. Now, their unit is filled with laughter and delicious smells, proving that meal prep can be a team sport. Who knew that nursing could foster not just healing but also culinary creativity?

These nurses show that with a little humor, creativity, and a dash of competition, meal prep can transform your approach to eating healthy. Whether you're whipping up a batch of chili like Sarah, mastering the art of stir-fry like Tom, perfecting energy balls like Jessica, or engaging in culinary battles like Mark and Liz, remember that you're not alone in this journey. The key is to embrace the chaos, find joy in the process, and fuel your body with the nourishment it deserves. After all, if we can survive the night shift, we can certainly conquer meal prep.

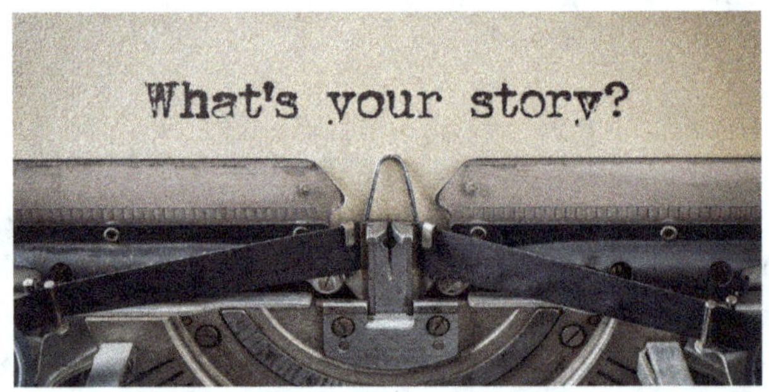

Lessons Learned: What We Wish We Knew Before We Started

When we first embarked on our meal prep journey, we had visions of perfectly organized Tupperware and Instagram-worthy salads. What we didn't anticipate was the sheer chaos that would ensue. It turns out that trying to chop vegetables while simultaneously dodging a cat who believes your cutting board is her personal runway is a recipe for disaster. If we could go back in time, we'd tell our past selves to invest in a solid pair of kitchen gloves and maybe a cat-proof kitchen. Lesson number one: a well-prepped kitchen is half the battle, and the other half is keeping the furry distractions at bay.

Next up on our list of things we wish we knew is that meal prepping isn't just about planning; it's about adaptability. Remember that time we thought we could make a week's worth of quinoa and broccoli and be the envy of all our colleagues? Yeah, that lasted about two days before we were staring down a bland, green mush that could double as a science experiment. We learned the hard way that variety is the spice of life—and the key to avoiding culinary boredom. So, stock up on some colorful produce and don't be afraid to switch things up. Your taste buds (and your sanity) will thank you.

Now let's talk about the budget. As nursing students or busy professionals, it's easy to fall into the trap of thinking that healthy meals must come with a hefty price tag. Spoiler alert: they don't! We wish we had known earlier that frozen fruits and veggies are just as nutritious as fresh ones and often come with a friendlier price tag. Plus, who doesn't love the idea of tossing some frozen spinach into a smoothie without worrying about it going bad? Our wallets are still recovering from those overpriced "fresh" avocados that turned out to be more rock than fruit.

And if we had a dollar for every time we said, "I'll just grab a snack from the vending machine," we'd be able to afford a personal chef. The truth is, when your shift is twelve hours long, the last thing you want is to rely on a chocolate bar for energy. We learned that having high-energy snacks on hand is essential for survival. Think protein-packed bites, easy-to-make energy balls, and maybe a few secret stashes of dark chocolate for those particularly rough shifts. Trust us, your fellow nurses will marvel at your snack game, and you'll avoid the dreaded post-vending machine crash.

Finally, let's wrap it up with a little wisdom about time management. We all know that time is a luxury we don't have as busy nurses. The irony is that meal prep is supposed to save you time, yet somehow it can end up being a whole weekend project. It's all about finding your rhythm. Maybe it's a Sunday afternoon or an hour on your day off. Whatever it is, block that time out and treat it like a sacred nursing shift—no interruptions allowed. The earlier you embrace the art of efficient meal prep, the more time you'll have to binge-watch your favorite shows or enjoy a well-deserved nap before your next shift.

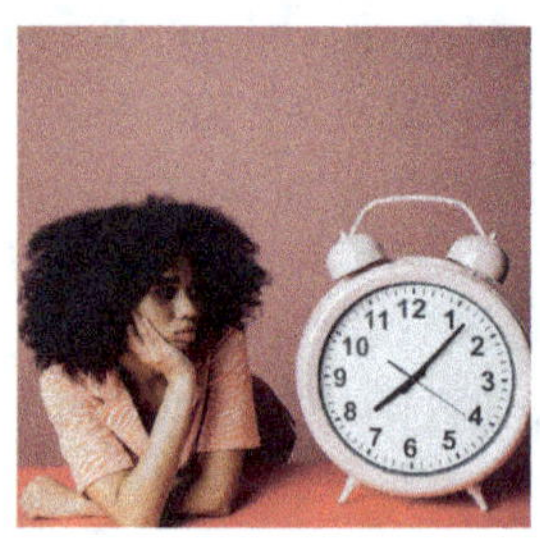

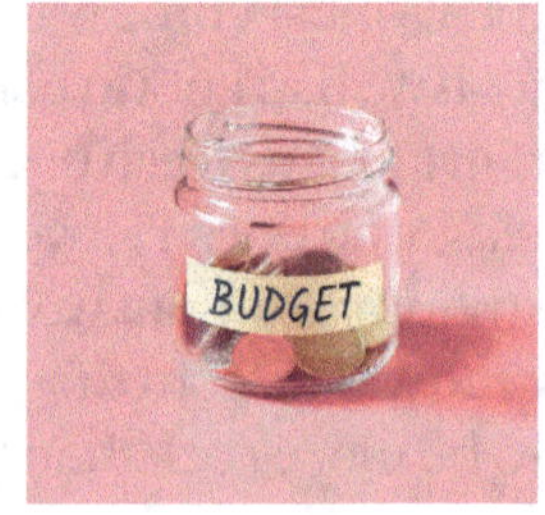

Celebrating Your Wins: How to Reward Yourself After a Successful Meal Prep Weekend

After a long weekend of chopping, stirring, and mastering the art of meal prep, it's time to celebrate your culinary conquests! Picture this: you've just finished assembling a week's worth of colorful, nutritious meals that would make even the pickiest of eaters swoon. You deserve a reward! But hold on, we're not talking about a three-tier chocolate cake (though, let's be real, that does sound tempting). Instead, let's get creative with some fun and lighthearted ways to pat yourself on the back without derailing your healthy eating mission.

First on the list? Dance it out! Yes, you heard me right. Crank up your favorite tunes and have a solo dance party in your kitchen. Nothing says "I'm a meal prep master" quite like a spontaneous dance break while you admire your neatly stacked containers. Just be careful not to spill any quinoa on the floor; you don't want to be slipping around like you're in a cooking show gone wrong. A little shimmy while you strut past your fridge will burn off a few calories and boost your mood, making you feel like the superstar chef you truly are.

Next, consider treating yourself to a "fancy" meal—at home! You've just spent hours prepping wholesome meals, so why not whip up something a little extra special for yourself? Think of it as a mini restaurant experience right in your kitchen. Light a candle, put on your comfiest pajamas, and serve your meal on your best dishes (or even some cute paper plates if you're feeling cheeky). Pair it with a .

refreshing beverage, and you've got yourself a date night with... yourself! Plus, it's a great way to show your tastebuds what they've been missing while you were busy being a meal-prepping whiz.

Now, let's not forget the power of a little pampering. After tirelessly chopping and stirring, your hands deserve some TLC. Treat yourself to a luxurious hand cream or a soothing soak in warm water infused with your favorite essential oils. As you relax, you can plan your next meal prep adventure or simply bask in the glory of your weekend achievements. Bonus points if you indulge in a face mask that makes you feel like a million bucks—because what's better than feeling fabulous while knowing you've got healthy meals prepped for the week ahead?

Finally, if you really want to take your celebration up a notch, gather your fellow nurse friends for a "Meal Prep Appreciation Night." Share your favorite recipes, swap tips, and enjoy a potluck of your creations. Who knew meal prep could spark such camaraderie? Plus, it's a chance to bond over the shared struggle of maintaining a healthy lifestyle amidst the chaos of night shifts and demanding schedules. Just remember to bring your sense of humor; laughter is the best seasoning, after all!

So, there you have it—celebrating your wins after a successful meal prep weekend doesn't have to be a chore. With a little creativity, some humor, and a sprinkle of indulgence, you can reward yourself in ways that make your busy nurse life a little brighter. Now, go ahead and dance, dine, pamper, and party your way into a week of healthy eating that you can truly savor!

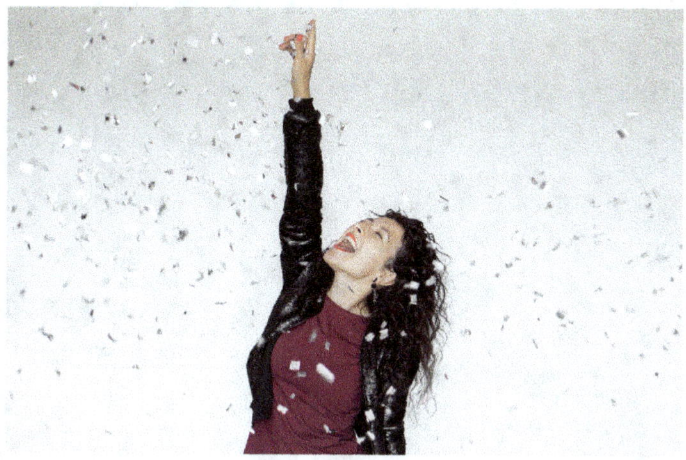

www.ingramcontent.com/pod-product-compliance
Lightning Source LLC
Chambersburg PA
CBHW050805250726

48653CB00006B/2091